PREFACE

There are no short cuts to the process of learning! The material on the following pages is not designed to provide the reader with an opportunity to escape from learning basic information that can only be obtained from textbooks. The purpose of this text is to encourage the reader to detect areas of weakness in his understanding of subject matter so that he may return to his texts for a more comprehensive review of the subject. Crossword puzzles are not designed to teach basic English; examination review books do not teach a basic understanding of the subject. However, the following pages will provide an interesting challenge to the student as well as an opportunity to improve his skills with multiple-choice examinations.

The completely referenced form of the question material is provided to facilitate the reader in checking his areas of weakness. Do not compromise by simply looking up the correct answers — the mature approach is to return to your textbook. The author has provided you with a time saving device in rapidly finding a source of information. While testing your memory be aware of the textbook as being the ultimate source of your fund of knowledge. References cited in the individual questions are listed on page 205.

The variations in test questions are offered to familiarize the reader with various types of National Board, State Board and School examinations in use today. The following test material will give you an opportunity to determine your ability to read, digest and comprehend the vast accumulation of available knowledge. Don't be discouraged if you are unable to achieve a perfect test score; indeed be stimulated to learn the material by referring to your textbooks. Successfully solving the problems in this text will surely give you satisfaction.

NERVOUS SYSTEM BASIC SCIENCES

1,500 MULTIPLE CHOICE QUESTIONS AND REFERENCED ANSWERS

Edited by

ROYCE L. MONTGOMERY, Ph.D.
Assistant Professor
Department of Anatomy
University of North Carolina
Chapel Hill, North Carolina

Contributors:

MICHAEL K. BERKUT, Ph.D.
Associate Professor
Department of Biochemistry

EDWARD L. HOGAN, M.D.
Associate Professor
Department of Medicine and Neurology

MARY C. SINGLETON, Ph.D.
Assistant Professor
Department of Anatomy

UNIVERSITY OF NORTH CAROLINA
CHAPEL HILL, NORTH CAROLINA

ALEXANDER A. FEDINEC, Ph.D.
Associate Professor
Department of Anatomy
University of Tennessee
Memphis, Tennessee

MEDICAL EXAMINATION PUBLISHING COMPANY, INC.
65-36 Fresh Meadow Lane
Flushing, New York 11365

Library of Congress
Catalog Card Number
72-77074

ISBN 0-87488-210-9

March 1972

PRINTED IN THE UNITED STATES OF AMERICA

TABLE OF CONTENTS

FOR EACH OF THE FOLLOWING MULTIPLE CHOICE QUESTIONS, SELECT THE MOST APPROPRIATE ANSWER(S):

1. LEPTOMENINX REFERS TO THE:
A. Dura mater
B. Dura mater and arachnoid
C. Pia and arachnoid
D. Superficial glial membrane
E. Periosteum
Ref. 7 - p. 12

2. THE SPINAL DURA EXTENDS FROM THE MARGINS OF THE FORAMEN MAGNUM TO THE LEVEL OF THE:
A. First lumbar vertebra
B. Third lumbar vertebra
C. First sacral vertebra
D. Second sacral vertebra
E. First coccygeal vertebra
Ref. 7 - p. 12

3. IN ADULTS THE SPINAL CORD USUALLY TERMINATES AT THE:
A. Upper border of the 12th thoracic vertebra
B. Lower border of the 1st lumbar vertebra
C. Upper border of the 4th lumbar vertebra
D. Level of 5th lumbar vertebra
E. End of sacral canal
Ref. 7 - p. 12

4. THE MIDDLE MENINGEAL ARTERY IS A BRANCH OF THE__________ ARTERY:
A. Deep temporal
B. Vertebral
C. Occipital
D. Frontal
E. Maxillary
Ref. 7 - p. 13

5. THE SPINAL CORD IS ANCHORED TO THE DURA MATER BY THE:
A. Coccygeal ligament
B. Ligamentum flavum
C. Anterior longitudinal ligament
D. Denticulate ligaments
E. Cauda equina
Ref. 7 - p. 15

6. ARACHNOID GRANULATIONS ARE:
A. Prolongations of pia-arachnoid
B. Prolongations of dura mater
C. Sites of fluid transfer from the venous sinuses to the subarachnoid space
D. Sites of cerebrospinal fluid formation
E. A pathological feature of the pia-arachnoid
Ref. 7 - p. 19

7. THE BULK OF THE CEREBROSPINAL FLUID IS FORMED BY:
A. Passive transport of Na^+ and Cl^- across the epithelial cells of the choroid plexus
B. Active transport of ions across the choroid plexus
C. Filtration from the capillary beds of pia-arachnoid
D. Secretion by arachnoid granulations
E. Filtration from the lymphatics of the meninges
Ref. 7 - p. 21

8. THE STRUCTURE WHICH DOES NOT STAIN AFTER INTRAVENOUS INJECTION OF VITAL DYES IS THE:
A. Pineal body
B. Pituitary gland
C. Area postrema
D. Choroid plexus
E. Cerebral cortex — Ref. 7 - p. 24

9. AT BIRTH THE TIP OF THE CONUS MEDULLARIS REACHES THE:
A. First lumbar vertebra
B. Second lumbar vertebra
C. Third lumbar vertebra
D. First sacral vertebra
E. Second sacral vertebra — Ref. 7 - p. 26

10. IN THE ADULT, THE 12-TH THORACIC SPINAL SEGMENT CORRESPONDS TO THE SPINOUS PROCESS OF VERTEBRA:
A. T-X
B. T-XII
C. L-I
D. L-II
E. L-III — Ref. 7 - p. 28

11. THE EXTERNAL FEATURES OF THE SPINAL CORD DO NOT INCLUDE THE:
A. Anterior median fissure
B. Posterior median sulcus
C. Posterior lateral sulcus
D. Posterior intermediate sulcus
E. Sulcus limitans — Ref. 7 - p. 29

12. FUNICULUS REFERS TO THE:
A. Gray matter
B. White matter
C. Anterior white commissure
D. Cortico-spinal tract
E. Fasciculus cuneatus — Ref. 7 - p. 29

13. ALL THE LISTED STRUCTURES ARE PARTS OF THE BRAIN STEM, EXCEPT THE:
A. Medulla
B. Pons
C. Midbrain
D. Cerebellum
E. Diencephalon — Ref. 7 - p. 30

14. THE FIBER BUNDLE CONNECTING CEREBELLUM AND MIDBRAIN IS THE:
A. Inferior cerebellar peduncle (restiform body)
B. Middle cerebellar peduncle (brachium pontis)
C. Superior cerebellar peduncle (brachium conjuctivum)
D. Internal capsule
E. Cerebral peduncle — Ref. 7 - p. 30

15. ALL THE LISTED FUNCTIONAL NERVE FIBERS ARE PART OF THE SPINAL NERVE, EXCEPT:
A. General somatic afferent (GSA)
B. General somatic efferent (GSE)
C. General visceral afferent (GVA)
D. General visceral efferent (GVE)
E. Special visceral afferent (SVA) Ref. 7 - p. 252

16. THE HYPOGLOSSAL NERVE (XII) EMERGES FROM THE MEDULLA THROUGH THE:
A. Anterior median fissure
B. Postolivary sulcus
C. Anterolateral (preolivary) sulcus
D. Sulcus limitans
E. Posteromedian sulcus Ref. 7 - p. 34

17. CEREBROSPINAL FLUID ESCAPES FROM THE VENTRICLES INTO THE SUBARACHNOID SPACE THROUGH THE:
A. Central canal
B. Cerebral aqueduct
C. Choroid plexus
D. Interventricular foramen
E. Foramina of Luschka and Magendie Ref. 7 - p. 35

18. THE DEPRESSION AT THE CAUDAL END OF THE RHOMBOID FOSSA IS CALLED THE:
A. Inferior fovea
B. Area postrema
C. Median eminence
D. Calamus scriptorius (obex)
E. Superior fovea Ref. 7 - p. 31

19. THE QUADRIGEMINAL PLATE IS PART OF THE:
A. Roof of the fourth ventricle
B. Medulla
C. Diencephalon
D. Midbrain tectum
E. Pontine tegmentum Ref. 7 - p. 39

20. THE POSTERIOR PERFORATED SUBSTANCE IS LOCATED IN THE AREA OF THE:
A. Lateral recess of fourth ventricle
B. Third ventricle
C. Olfactory trigone
D. Interpeduncular fossa
E. Inferior medullary velum Ref. 7 - p. 39

21. THE EPITHALAMUS INCLUDES THE:
A. Pulvinar
B. Mammillary body
C. Tuber cinereum
D. Geniculate bodies
E. Pineal body Ref. 7 - p. 39

22. THE THIRD VENTRICLE COMMUNICATES WITH THE FOURTH VENTRICLE BY THE:
A. Interventricular foramen
B. Central canal
C. Foramen of Luschka
D. Foramen of Magendie
E. Cerebral aqueduct — Ref. 7 - p. 41

23. THE BASAL GANGLIA DO NOT INCLUDE THE:
A. Caudate nuclei
B. Lenticular nuclei
C. Amygdaloid nuclei
D. Claustrum
E. Thalamus — Ref. 7 - p. 42

24. CORPUS STRIATUM REFERS TO THE:
A. Caudate and lenticular nuclei
B. Caudate and anterior thalamic nuclei
C. Optic radiations
D. Globus pallidus and putamen
E. Geniculate bodies — Ref. 7 - p. 42

25. TENTORIUM CEREBELLI OCCUPIES THE:
A. Longitudinal fissure
B. Lateral sulcus
C. Central sulcus
D. Transverse fissure
E. Insula — Ref. 7 - p. 44

26. THE PRECENTRAL GYRUS IS PART OF THE:
A. Frontal lobe
B. Parietal lobe
C. Occipital lobe
D. Temporal lobe
E. Cerebellum — Ref. 7 - p. 45

27. THE ANGULAR GYRUS IS PART OF THE:
A. Cerebellum
B. Frontal lobe
C. Parietal lobe
D. Occipital lobe
E. Temporal lobe — Ref. 7 - p. 45

28. THE INSULA (ISLAND OF REIL) LIES IN THE:
A. Hippocampal sulcus
B. Longitudinal fissure
C. Transverse fissure
D. Central sulcus
E. Lateral sulcus — Ref. 7 - p. 46

29. THE LONGITUDINAL SULCUS DIVIDES THE INSULA INTO THE GYRI:
A. Brevis and longus
B. Precentral and postcentral
C. Pars triangularis and pars opercularis of inferior frontal gyrus
D. Transverse temporal and supramarginal
E. Superior temporal and middle temporal
Ref. 7 - p. 46

30. THE TERMS SPLENIUM, GENU AND ROSTRUM REFER TO THE:
A. Fornix
B. Caudate nucleus
C. Stria terminalis
D. Internal capsule
E. Corpus callosum Ref. 7 - p. 48

31. THE CALLOSAL SULCUS CONTINUES CAUDALLY AS THE:
A. Sulcus cinguli
B. Marginal sulcus
C. Paracentral sulcus
D. Hippocampal sulcus
E. Parieto-occipital sulcus Ref. 7 - p. 49

32. THE CUNEUS AND PRECUNEUS ARE SEPARATED BY THE__________ SULCUS:
A. Parieto-occipital
B. Subparietal
C. Cingulate
D. Intra-parietal
E. Collateral Ref. 7 - p. 50

33. THE INTERNAL CAPSULE IS COMPOSED OF NERVE FIBERS CLASSIFIED AS:
A. Projectional
B. Short associational
C. Commissural
D. Arcuate
E. Long associational Ref. 7 - p. 51

34. ALL THE FOLLOWING FIBERS FORM THE INTERNAL CAPSULE, <u>EXCEPT</u> THE:
A. Corticospinal
B. Corticobulbar
C. Frontopontine
D. Temporo-parietopontine
E. Occipito-frontal Ref. 7 - p. 52

35. THE__________FIBRE BUNDLE PROJECTS FROM THE HIPPOCAMPUS TO THE HYPOTHALAMUS:
A. Uncinate fasciculus
B. Superior longitudinal fasciculus
C. Inferior occipitofrontal fasciculus
D. Inferior longitudinal fasciculus
E. Fornix Ref. 7 - p. 56

36. IDENTIFY THE TERM NOT ASSOCIATED WITH THE LATERAL VENTRICLES:
A. Anterior or frontal horn
B. Collateral trigone
C. Posterior or occipital horn
D. Calcar avis
E. Lateral recess Ref. 7 - p. 57

37. THE ANTERIOR SPINAL ARTERY IS A BRANCH OF THE__________ ARTERY:
A. Posterior inferior cerebellar
B. Superior cerebellar
C. Thoracic aorta
D. Internal carotid
E. Vertebral Ref. 7 - p. 60

38. THE BLOOD SUPPLY OF THE SPINAL CORD MAY BE JEOPARDIZED IN REGIONS WHERE ITS ARTERIAL SUPPLY IS DERIVED FROM TWO DIFFERENT SOURCES. SUCH AN AREA INCLUDES SPINAL SEGMENTS:
A. C_1-C_4
B. C_4-C_8
C. T_1-T_4
D. T_8-T_{12}
E. S_1-S_3 Ref. 7 - p. 61

39. THE ANTERIOR CHOROIDAL ARTERY USUALLY ARISES FROM THE__________ARTERY:
A. Internal carotid
B. Vertebral
C. Anterior communicating
D. Anterior cerebral
E. Posterior cerebral Ref. 7 - p. 63

40. THE VERTEBRAL ARTERY ENTERS THE CRANIAL FOSSA THROUGH THE:
A. Foramen ovale
B. Foramen spinosum
C. Jugular foramen
D. Foramen cecum
E. Foramen magnum Ref. 7 - p. 63

41. IDENTIFY THE ARTERY WHICH DOES NOT PARTICIPATE IN FORMATION OF THE CEREBRAL ARTERIAL CIRCLE (OF WILLIS):
A. Anterior and posterior communicating
B. Anterior cerebral
C. Middle cerebral
D. Posterior cerebral
E. Vertebral Ref. 7 - p. 63

42. THE HEAD OF THE CAUDATE NUCLEUS, THE INTERNAL CAPSULE AND THE PUTAMEN ARE SUPPLIED BY THE__________ARTERY:
A. Medial striate (of Huebner)
B. Anterior choroidal
C. Posterior choroidal
D. Anteromedial branches of anterior cerebral
E. Posteromedial branches of the posterior cerebral
Ref. 7 - p. 66

43. THE MOTOR AND PREMOTOR AREAS AND THE SOMESTHETIC AND AUDITORY PROJECTION AREAS ARE SUPPLIED BY THE__________ ARTERY:
A. Anterior cerebral
B. Middle cerebral
C. Posterior cerebral
D. Medial striate
E. Lateral striate Ref. 7 - p. 68

44. WITH THE EXCEPTION OF THE__________AREA THE ANTERIOR CHOROIDAL ARTERY SUPPLIES THE:
A. Hippocampal formation
B. Globus pallidus
C. Internal capsule
D. Amygdaloid nucleus
E. Hypothalamus Ref. 7 - p. 72

45. THE BULBAR BRANCHES OF THE VERTEBRAL ARTERY SUPPLY THE:
A. Gracilis nucleus
B. Cuneate nucleus
C. Inferior cerebellar peduncle
D. Hypoglossal nucleus
E. Vestibular nuclei Ref. 7 - p. 74

46. IDENTIFY THE ARTERY WHICH IS NOT A BRANCH OF THE BASILAR ARTERY:
A. Anterior inferior cerebellar
B. Labyrinthine
C. Paramedian and circumferential rami
D. Superior cerebellar
E. Posterior inferior cerebellar Ref. 7 - p. 74

47. THE__________SINUS EXTENDS FROM THE FORAMEN CECUM TO THE INTERNAL OCCIPITAL PROTUBERANCE:
A. Superior sagittal
B. Inferior sagittal
C. Sinus rectus
D. Sphenoparietal
E. Superior petrosal Ref. 7 - p. 81

48. THE DURA MATER OF THE POSTERIOR CRANIAL FOSSA IS SUPPLIED BY THE_________ARTERY:
A. Anterior meningeal
B. Middle meningeal
C. Meningeal branches of occipital, vertebral and ascending pharyngeal
D. Posterior cerebral
E. Posterior superior cerebellar Ref. 7 - p. 80

49. THE CAVERNOUS SINUS COMMUNICATES WITH THE_________SINUS:
A. Rectus
B. Transverse
C. Sigmoid
D. Superior sagittal
E. Superior petrosal Ref. 7 - p. 82

50. THE PARIETAL FORAMEN TRANSMITS THE_________VEIN:
A. Cerebral
B. Meningeal
C. Diploic
D. Emissary
E. Jugular Ref. 7 - p. 83

51. THE_________VEIN DOES NOT DRAIN INTO THE INTERNAL CEREBRAL VEIN:
A. Thalamostriate
B. Choroidal
C. Septal
D. Epithalamic
E. Inferior cerebral Ref. 7 - p. 86

52. THE ALAR PLATES OF THE EMBRYONIC SPINAL CORD DIFFERENTIATE INTO THE:
A. Dorsal root ganglia
B. Autonomic ganglia
C. Sensory horns (posterior)
D. Motor horns (ventral)
E. Intermediolateral cell column Ref. 7 - p. 92

53. THE OLIGODENDROGLIA ARE DERIVED FROM THE:
A. Primitive spongioblasts
B. Apolar neuroblasts
C. Medulloblasts
D. Astroblasts
E. Microglia Ref. 7 - p. 93

54. UNIPOLAR NEURONES ARE FOUND IN THE:
A. Ciliary ganglia
B. Otic ganglia
C. Superior cervical ganglia
D. Dorsal root ganglia
E. Celiac ganglion Ref. 7 - p. 96

55. THE PROSENCEPHALON DIFFERENTIATES INTO THE:
A. Myelencephalon
B. Metencephalon
C. Mesencephalon
D. Rhombencephalon
E. Telencephalon and Diencephalon Ref. 7 - p. 98

56. THE CEREBELLUM DEVELOPS FROM THE:
A. Telencephalon
B. Diencephalon
C. Mesencephalon
D. Metencephalon
E. Myelencephalon Ref. 7 - p. 100

57. DEVELOPMENTALLY THE OPTIC NERVES REMAIN ASSOCIATED WITH THE:
A. Telencephalon
B. Diencephalon
C. Mesencephalon
D. Metencephalon
E. Myelencephalon Ref. 7 - p. 102

58. THE COMMISSURAL FIBERS OF THE CORPUS CALLOSUM DEVELOP IN THE:
A. Roof of the mesencephalon
B. Lamina terminalis
C. Telencephalon
D. Mesencephalon
E. Metencephalon Ref. 7 - p. 106

59. CHROMOPHIL SUBSTANCE (MASSES OF ENDOPLASMIC RETICULUM) FORM:
A. Nissl Bodies
B. The Centrosome
C. Mitochondria
D. The Golgi Apparatus
E. The Nucleolus Ref. 7 - p. 121

60. SCHWANN CELLS ORIGINATE FROM:
A. Primitive spongioblasts
B. Medulloblasts
C. Ectoderm
D. Mesoderm
E. Entoderm Ref. 7 - p. 130

61. THE MYELIN SHEATH OF THE PERIPHERAL NERVE IS FORMED BY:
A. Fibroblasts
B. Spongioblasts
C. Macrophages
D. Oligodendroglia
E. Schwann cells Ref. 7 - p. 127

62. THE PERINEURAL EPITHELIUM IS PART OF THE:
A. Epineurium
B. Outermost layers of perineurium
C. Innermost layers of perineurium
D. Endoneurium
E. Myelin sheath Ref. 7 - p. 132

63. MYELINATED FIBERS HAVING A DIAMETER OF 1 TO 20 MICRA AND A CONDUCTION RATE OF 5 TO 120 METERS ARE CLASSIFIED AS__________FIBERS:
A. Gamma
B. Autonomic
C. "A"
D. "B"
E. "C" Ref. 7 - p. 135

64. TYPE "B" FIBERS ARE MAINLY ASSOCIATED WITH__________ INNERVATION:
A. Muscular
B. Cutaneous
C. Somatic
D. Visceral
E. Proprioceptive Ref. 7 - p. 135

65. THE GEMMULES ARE:
A. Axoaxonic synapses
B. Axosomatic synapses
C. Axodendritic synapses
D. Neuropodia
E. Spiny projections on dendrites Ref. 7 - p. 137

66. SOME OF THE WAYS IN WHICH CONDUCTION ACROSS THE SYNAPSE DIFFERS FROM THAT IN A NERVE FIBER:
A. Conduction is slower
B. Conduction is faster
C. Response may persist after cessation of the stimulus
D. Less fatigability
E. Greater fatigability Ref. 7 - p. 139

67. THE SIMPLEST SEGMENTAL REFLEX REQUIRES A CHAIN OF AT LEAST__________NEURONS:
A. 2
B. 4
C. 7
D. 1
E. 5 Ref. 7 - p. 136

68. B TYPE FIBERS ARE MAINLY ASSOCIATED WITH__________ INNERVATION:
A. Somatic
B. Visceral
C. Skeletal muscle
D. Cardiac muscle
E. Smooth muscle Ref. 7 - p. 135

69. ALL THE FOLLOWING CELLS ARE NEUROGLIA, <u>EXCEPT</u>:
A. Oligodendrocytes
B. Fibrous and protoplasmic astrocytes
C. Microglia
D. Ependyma
E. Pineal cells Ref. 7 - p. 149

70. THE PERINEURONAL SATELLITE CELLS ARE CLASSIFIED AS:
A. Oligodendroglia
B. Fibrous astrocytes
C. Microglia
D. Protoplasmic astrocytes
E. Golgi type II Ref. 7 - p. 151

71. INCLUDED AMONG THE FUNCTIONS OF OLIGODENDROGLIA IS:
A. Participation as intermediary in neuronal metabolism
B. Participation in unidirectional impulse conduction
C. Secretion of cerebrospinal fluid
D. Collagen formation
E. Phagocytosis Ref. 7 - p. 151

72. THE FUNCTIONS OF ASTROCYTES DO NOT INCLUDE:
A. Participation in transport of metabolites between blood and neurones
B. Reaction to injury by swelling
C. Myelin formation
D. Packing of neuropil
E. Formation of perivascular end feet Ref. 7 - p. 152

73. ALL OF THE FOLLOWING STATEMENTS ARE TRUE ABOUT MICROGLIA, <u>EXCEPT</u>:
A. Mesodermal origin
B. Source of macrophages
C. Found in the gray matter
D. Irregular perykaryon and few thick processes
E. Rounded nucleus Ref. 7 - p. 155

74. ALL OF THE FOLLOWING STATEMENTS ARE TRUE ABOUT THE EPENDYMAL CELLS, <u>EXCEPT</u>:
A. Line the central canal of the spinal cord and the ventricles of the brain
B. In adult, form a single layer of cuboidal cells
C. Have secretory and absorptive functions
D. Participate in formation of brain-cerebrospinal fluid barrier
E. Line the arachnoid villi Ref. 7 - p. 159

75. IN THE ADULT THE CHOROIDAL EPITHELIUM CONSISTS OF:
A. Squamous cells
B. Tall columnar cells
C. Low cuboidal cells
D. Absorptive cells only
E. Phagocytic cells Ref. 7 - p. 161

76. THE NERVE CELLS OF THE ADULT DORSAL ROOT GANGLIA ARE:
A. Pseudounipolar
B. Bipolar
C. Large multipolar
D. Small multipolar
E. Pseudobipolar Ref. 7 - p. 166

77. THE SATELLITE CELLS IN THE DORSAL ROOT GANGLIA ARE DERIVED FROM:
A. Neural crest
B. Basal plate
C. Schwann cells
D. Ependymal cells
E. Fibroblast cells Ref. 7 - p. 167

78. THE FOLLOWING SENSORY MODALITIES ARE ASSOCIATED WITH THE EXTEROCEPTORS, EXCEPT:
A. Touch
B. Light pressure
C. Smell
D. Sight
E. Sensation of position Ref. 7 - p. 174

79. INTEROCEPTORS RECEIVE AND TRANSMIT SENSORY IMPULSES THAT ARE:
A. Poorly localized
B. Sharply localized
C. Associated with hearing
D. Associated with sight
E. Temperature related Ref. 7 - p. 175

80. DISCRIMINATIVE SENSIBILITY ACCURATELY LOCALIZES THE STIMULUS. IT IS ALSO KNOWN AS THE __________ SENSIBILITY:
A. Protopathic
B. Epicritic
C. Visceral
D. Interoceptive
E. Thalamic Ref. 7 - p. 175

81. THE PAIN RECEPTORS ARE THE:
A. Corpuscles of Meissner
B. Pacinian corpuscles
C. Golgi-Mazzoni corpuscles
D. Organs of Golgi
E. Free nerve endings Ref. 7 - p. 176

82. THE SENSORY RECEPTOR RESPONDING TO CHANGES IN LOCAL BLOOD SUPPLY, DEFORMATION AND VIBRATORY STIMULI IS THE:
A. Meissner's corpuscle
B. Pacinian corpuscle
C. Golgi-Mazzoni corpuscle
D. End bulb of Krause
E. Free nerve ending Ref. 7 - p. 181

83. THE NEUROMUSCULAR SPINDLE CONSISTS OF:
A. Tendon fascicles surrounded by a connective tissue capsule
B. Smooth muscle fibers surrounded by a connective tissue capsule
C. Striated muscle fibers surrounded by a connective tissue capsule
D. Layers of connective lamellae of flattened cells with semifluid substance in the center
E. Diffuse arborization of nerve endings among striated muscle fibers
Ref. 7 - p. 182

84. TOUCH IS REPRESENTED BY THE ENDINGS IN WHICH OF THE FOLLOWING?:
A. Hair follicles
B. Meissner's corpuscles
C. End bulbs of Krause
D. Corpuscles of Pacini
E. Tactile discs
Ref. 7 - p. 188

85. THE POSTGANGLIONIC CELL BODIES OF AXONS INNERVATING CARDIAC MUSCLE ARE LOCATED IN THE:
A. Ventral horn of the spinal cord
B. Dorsal horn of the spinal cord
C. Dorsal root ganglia
D. Medulla
E. Autonomic ganglia
Ref. 7 - p. 189

86. THE MOTOR ENDING ON A SKELETAL MUSCLE FIBER SHOWS:
A. Nerve terminals within the sarcoplasm of the muscle fiber
B. Nerve terminals in the junction folds
C. Absence of mitochondria
D. Presence of a synaptic gutter
Ref. 7 - p. 191

87. THE AUTONOMIC FIBERS WHICH SUPPLY VISCERAL MUSCLE (SMOOTH MUSCLE) TERMINATE AS:
A. Motor end plates similar to those of skeletal muscle
B. Encapsulated end organs
C. Small thickenings or delicate loops on the surface of the muscle fibers
D. Ovoid bodies formed by epitheloid cells and a connective tissue capsule
E. Concave neurofibrillar discs
Ref. 7 - p. 193

88. DUE TO DEVELOPMENTAL MIGRATION OF METAMERES INTO THE EXTREMITY, THE SEQUENCE OF DERMATOMES IN THE NECK AND TRUNK IS AS FOLLOWS:
A. C3 to C7
B. C4 to C8
C. C4 to T2
D. C7 to T2
E. C8 to T3
Ref. 7 - p. 193

89. THE BICEPS TENDON REFLEX (FLEXION OF FOREARM ON PERCUSSION OF BICEPS TENDON) INVOLVES SPINAL SEGMENTS:
A. C3-4
B. C4
C. C5-6
D. C7-T1
E. C5-T1
Ref. 7 - p. 199

90. THE CREMASTERIC REFLEX (ELEVATION OF SCROTUM ON STROKING OF INNER THIGH) INVOLVES SPINAL SEGMENTS:
A. C3-4
B. C5-6
C. T1-10
D. T12-L2
E. S1-3
Ref. 7 - p. 199

91. THE PATELLAR TENDON REFLEX OR KNEE JERK (EXTENSION OF LEG ON PERCUSSION OF PATELLAR LIGAMENT) INVOLVES SPINAL SEGMENTS:
A. C5-T1
B. T1-T10
C. L2-L4
D. L1-S2
E. S1-S3
Ref. 7 - p. 199

92. THE CERVICAL PLEXUS IS FORMED BY THE__________SPINAL NERVES:
A. Dorsal rami of Cl-4
B. Ventral rami of Cl-4
C. Dorsal rami of C5-T1
D. Ventral rami of C5-T1
E. Ventral rami of Cl-3
Ref. 7 - p. 201

93. THE PHRENIC NERVE WHICH SUPPLIES THE DIAPHRAGM ORIGINATES FROM SPINAL SEGMENTS:
A. Cl-3
B. C3-5
C. C5-T1
D. T1-7
E. T5-10
Ref. 7 - p. 201

94. THE ACCESSORY NERVE (N. XI) SUPPLIES MOTOR FIBERS TO THE__________MUSCLE:
A. Temporal
B. Occipital
C. Platysma
D. Sternohyoid
E. Trapezius
Ref. 7 - p. 201

95. THE BRACHIAL PLEXUS IS FORMED BY THE:
A. Dorsal and ventral rami of C-5 nerves
B. Dorsal and ventral rami of C4-T2 nerves
C. Dorsal rami of C4-T1 nerves
D. Ventral rami of C4-T1 nerves
E. Ventral rami of T1-4 nerves
Ref. 7 - p. 202

96. THE MEDIAN NERVE SUPPLIES:
A. Coracobrachialis and brachialis
B. Flexor carpi ulnaris and ulnar head of flexor digitorum profundus
C. Triceps and anconeus
D. The thenar muscles
E. All flexors of the forearm
Ref. 7 - p. 206

97. THE LUMBOSACRAL PLEXUS IS FORMED BY THE SPINAL NERVES:
A. L1-S3
B. T12-S3
C. T10-L5
D. T10-S3
E. L3-S1
Ref. 7 - p. 208

98. THE SUPERIOR GLUTEAL NERVE IS DISTRIBUTED TO WHICH OF THE FOLLOWING MUSCLES?:
A. Gluteus medius
B. Gluteus minimus
C. Adductor longus
D. Adductor brevis
E. Gluteus maximus
Ref. 7 - p. 212

99. THE __________ NERVE SUPPLIES THE LATERAL AND ANTERIOR MUSCLES OF THE LEG AND THE DORSAL MUSCLES OF THE FOOT:
A. Lateral femoral cutaneous
B. Tibial
C. Common peroneal
D. Superior gluteal
E. Posterior femoral cutaneous
Ref. 7 - p. 213

100. AGGREGATIONS OF AUTONOMIC CELLS IN THE MESENTERIC PLEXUS ARE CLASSIFIED AS __________ GANGLIA:
A. Paravertebral
B. Prevertebral
C. Terminal
D. Intramural
E. Dorsal root
Ref. 7 - p. 217

101. THE SPINAL ORIGIN OF AUTONOMIC NERVE FIBERS FORMING THE WHITE RAMI COMMUNICANTES IS:
A. C1-S3
B. C8-S3
C. T1-S3
D. T1-L3
E. S2-3
Ref. 7 - p. 219

102. THE WHITE RAMI COMMUNICANTES CONNECT:
A. The superior cervical ganglion with the C1-4 nerves
B. Spinal cord segments C1-4 with the superior cervical ganglion
C. Sympathetic chain ganglia with all the spinal nerves
D. All spinal cord segments with the sympathetic chain ganglia
E. Spinal cord segments T1 to L3 with all sympathetic chain ganglia
Ref. 7 - p. 219

103. SYMPATHETIC POSTGANGLIONIC FIBERS SUPPLYING THE DILATOR MUSCLE OF THE IRIS ARISE FROM THE __________ GANGLION:
A. Ciliary
B. Pterygopalatine
C. Otic
D. Celiac
E. Superior cervical
Ref. 7 - p. 219

104. THE GREATER SPLANCHNIC NERVE ARISES BY ROOTS FROM SYMPATHETIC CHAIN GANGLIA __________:
A. S2-3
B. T1-5
C. T5-9
D. T10-L3
E. C8-L3
Ref. 7 - p. 221

105. THE PREGANGLIONIC CELL BODIES CONCERNED WITH THE INNERVATION OF THE HEART ARE LOCATED IN SPINAL CORD SEGMENTS:
A. C1-4
B. C5-8
C. T1-5
D. T6-12
E. L1-5
Ref. 7 - p. 221

106. THE PARASYMPATHETIC INNERVATION OF THE URINARY BLADDER ORIGINATES IN SPINAL CORD SEGMENTS:
A. T1-5
B. T6-12
C. L2-4
D. S2-4
E. T5-9
Ref. 7 - p. 221

107. THE SWEAT GLANDS OF THE FACE RECEIVE POSTGANGLIONIC NERVE FIBERS FROM THE__________SYMPATHETIC GANGLION:
A. Submandibular
B. Pterygopalatine
C. Otic
D. Upper thoracic
E. Superior cervical
Ref. 7 - p. 221

108. THE CELL BODIES OF THE VISCERAL AFFERENT FIBERS INNERVATING THE LUNGS ARE LOCATED IN THE__________SENSORY GANGLION:
A. Inferior vagal
B. Superior vagal
C. Inferior glossopharyngeal
D. Superior glossopharyngeal
E. Terminal plexus of pulmonary
Ref. 7 - p. 224

109. THE__________GANGLION IS CHARACTERIZED BY MULTIPOLAR NEURONS WITH ECCENTRIC NUCLEI, AND INTRA AND EXTRA CAPSULAR DENDRITIC ARBORIZATIONS:
A. Superior vagal
B. Trigeminal
C. Geniculate
D. Dorsal root
E. Autonomic
Ref. 7 - p. 224

110. "CHOLINERGIC" SYMPATHETIC POSTGANGLIONIC FIBERS INNERVATE:
A. Sweat glands
B. Parotid gland
C. Intestinal glands
D. Smooth muscle
E. Cardiac muscle
Ref. 7 - p. 226

111. ALL THE FOLLOWING FUNCTIONS OF THE PARASYMPATHETIC NERVOUS SYSTEM ARE CORRECT, EXCEPT:
A. Pupillary constriction (miosis)
B. Bronchial dilatation
C. Decrease of heart rate
D. Stimulation of gastrointestinal motility and secretion
E. Relaxation of gastrointestinal sphincters
Ref. 7 - p. 227

112. THE FUNCTIONS OF THE SYMPATHETIC NERVOUS SYSTEM DO NOT INCLUDE:
A. Stimulation of secretion of adrenal medulla
B. Constriction of ductus deferens
C. Reduction in volume of salivary secretion
D. Stimulation of secretion of sweat glands
E. Stimulation of gastrointestinal mobility
Ref. 7 - p. 227

113. THE TARSAL MUSCLE OF THE EYELID IS INNERVATED BY WHICH OF THE FOLLOWING NERVES?:

A. Sympathetics
B. Oculomotor
C. Trochlear
D. Abducens
E. Trigeminal

Ref. 7 - p. 232

114. THE ACTIVITIES OF THE PARASYMPATHETIC NERVOUS SYSTEM DO NOT INCLUDE:

A. Restoration and conservation of bodily energy
B. Mobilization of bodily reserves during emergencies
C. Initiation of response primarily by internal changes in the viscera
D. A discrete and limited effect to the portion stimulated
E. Release of acetylcholine by postganglionic fibers

Ref. 7 - p. 231

115. THE SACRAL SPINAL CORD SEGMENTS ARE CHARACTERIZED BY:

A. Oval shape
B. Predominance of white over gray matter
C. Pronounced intermediolateral cell columns
D. Presence of posterior intermediate septum
E. Thick quadrangular appearance of the gray matter

Ref. 7 - p. 238

116. THE CERVICAL SPINAL CORD SEGMENTS ARE CHARACTERIZED BY:

A. Pronounced intermediolateral nucleus
B. Predominance of gray over white matter
C. Presence of fasciculus gracilis and cuneatus
D. Small ventral and large dorsal gray horns
E. Cervical enlargement at segments C2-5

Ref. 7 - p. 239

117. THE CHARACTERISTICS OF NUCLEUS DORSALIS (OF CLARKE) INCLUDE ALL THE FOLLOWING FEATURES, EXCEPT:

A. Location at the mesial surface of the posterior horns
B. Extend from C8 to L3
C. Prominence in segments T10-12
D. Eccentrically placed nucleus in cells
E. Axons leaving via ventral roots

Ref. 7 - p. 240

118. THE SPINAL ROOT CELLS CONSTITUTE THE __________ NEURONS:

A. Substantia gelatinosa
B. Internuncial
C. Commissural
D. Association
E. Somatic and visceral efferent

Ref. 7 - p. 242

119. ACCORDING TO REXED'S CYTOARCHITECTONIC ORGANIZATION OF THE SPINAL GRAY MATTER, THE ALPHA NEURONS ARE LOCATED IN LAMINA:

A. I
B. II
C. III
D. V
E. IX

Ref. 7 - p. 246

120. THE SOMATIC EFFERENT NEURONS WHICH INNERVATE THE SHORT AND LONG MUSCLES ATTACHED TO THE AXIAL SKELETON FORM THE_________NUCLEAR GROUP IN THE SPINAL CORD:
A. Medial
B. Anterolateral
C. Posterolateral
D. Anterior
E. Retroposterolateral
Ref. 7 - p. 247

121. THE "RENSHAW" CELLS:
A. Are found in the reticular formation of the medulla
B. Receive synaptic terminals from the recurrent axon collaterals of large anterior horn cells
C. Give origin to axons forming the ventral spino-cerebellar tract
D. Supply the intrafusal fibers of the neuromuscular spindle
E. Are intimately related to axons of spinal white matter
Ref. 7 - p. 247

122. THE POSTERIOR HORN DOES NOT INCLUDE THE_________NUCLEAR GROUP:
A. Posteromarginal
B. Substantia gelatinosa
C. Proprius cornu posterior
D. Dorsalis (of Clarke)
E. Posterolateral of lateral group
Ref. 7 - p. 248

123. THE LATERAL BUNDLE OF THE DORSAL ROOT FIBERS ENTERING THE SPINAL CORD CONVEYS IMPULSES FROM THE:
A. Neuroepithelial cells
B. Neuromascular spindles
C. Large encapsulated somatic receptors
D. Neuro tendinous organs
E. Free nerve endings
Ref. 7 - p. 254

124. CLARKE'S NUCLEUS RECEIVES FIBERS FROM:
A. All spinal roots
B. All spinal roots except cervical roots
C. All thoracic and upper lumbar roots
D. S2-4 roots
E. Column cells only
Ref. 7 - p. 256

125. THE FASCICULUS GRACILIS CONSISTS OF:
A. Ascending root fibers from the upper thoracic and cervical ganglia
B. Descending fibers from cells of nucleus gracilis
C. Ascending root fibers from the sacral lumbar and lower thoracic ganglia
D. Ascending fibers from cells of nucleus proprius dorsalis
E. Ascending fibers from cells of nucleus dorsalis
Ref. 7 - p. 259

126. THE CHAIN OF NEURONES WHICH CONVEY TOUCH, PRESSURE AND KINESTHESIS ARE RELATED TO ALL THE FOLLOWING NERVE FIBERS, EXCEPT:
A. Central processes of dorsal root ganglia terminating in nucleus gracilis and cuneatus
B. Central processes of dorsal root ganglia terminating in nucleus dorsalis
C. Axons of nucleus gracilis and cuneatus terminating in the contralateral thalamus
D. Axons of posterolateral nucleus of the thalamus terminating in the sensory cortex
E. Axons of nucleus gracilis and cuneatus forming the internal arcuate fibers and medial lemniscus Ref. 7 - p. 259

127. THE END ORGANS INVOLVED IN PERCEPTION OF VIBRATORY SENSE PROBABLY ARE:
A. Free nerve endings
B. End bulbs of Krause
C. Pacinian corpuscles
D. Golgi-Mazzoni corpuscle
E. Meissner's corpuscle Ref. 7 - p. 261

128. ALL OF THE STATEMENTS BELOW CONCERNING THE DISTRIBUTION OF THE ANTERIOR SPINOTHALAMIC TRACT FIBERS ARE TRUE, EXCEPT:
A. Cross in the anterior commissure
B. Are arranged somatotopically, the caudal spinal segments being represented in the lateral part of the tract
C. In the medulla, pass adjacent to the lateral spinothalamic tract
D. In the upper pons, pass adjacent to the medial lemniscus
E. Terminate in the ventral posteromedial nucleus of the thalamus
Ref. 7 - p. 264

129. THE LATERAL SPINOTHALAMIC TRACT TRANSMITS IMPULSES OF__________TO HIGHER LEVELS OF THE NEURAXIS:
A. Light touch
B. Pressure
C. Sense of position and movement
D. Pain and temperature
E. Two point discrimination Ref. 7 - p. 265

130. THE CELLS OF ORIGIN (NEURON II) OF AXONS FORMING THE LATERAL SPINOTHALAMIC TRACT ARE LOCATED IN REXED'S LAMINAE__________:
A. I and II
B. III, IV and V
C. IV and V
D. VI, VII, VIII
E. IX Ref. 7 - p. 265

131. THE AXONS OF SPINAL NEURONS (NEURON II) FORMING THE LATERAL SPINOTHALAMIC TRACT CROSS IN THE:
A. Dorsal white commissure of the same spinal segment
B. Dorsal gray commissure of the same and adjacent spinal segments
C. Ventral white commissure of the same and adjacent spinal segments
D. Ventral gray commissure of the same spinal segment
E. Ventral white commissure of adjacent 4-5 spinal segments above the level of origin Ref. 7 - p. 265

132. THE FIBERS OF THE LATERAL SPINOTHALAMIC TRACT SHOW THE FOLLOWING SEGMENTAL ARRANGEMENT AT SPINAL LEVEL C-8:
A. The most lateral and posterior fibers represent the lowest portion of the body
B. The most medial and anterior fibers represent the lowest portion of the body
C. The most lateral and posterior fibers represent the upper extremities and neck
D. The posterior fibers conduct pain
E. The anterior fibers conduct thermal sense
Ref. 7 - p. 265

133. FIBERS OF THE SPINOTECTAL TRACT ASCEND IN THE SPINAL CORD AND BRAIN STEM IN CLOSE ASSOCIATION WITH WHICH OF THE FOLLOWING?:
A. Fasciculus gracilis
B. Lateral spinothalamic tract
C. Dorsal spinocerebellar tract
D. Ventral spinocerebellar tract
E. Clarke's column Ref. 7 - p. 271

134. THE FIBERS FORMING THE SPINOTECTAL TRACT CONDUCT:
A. Nociceptive impulses from the opposite side of the body
B. Positional sense from the opposite side of the body
C. Nociceptive impulses to superior colliculus
D. Positional sense to cerebellum
E. Two-point discrimination to thalamus
Ref. 7 - p. 269

135. THE POSTERIOR SPINOCEREBELLAR TRACT ORIGINATES IN THE CELLS OF:
A. Lamina I and II of Rexed
B. Intermediolateral cell column
C. Dorsal nucleus of Clarke
D. Anteromedial nucleus of all spinal segments
E. Posterolateral nucleus of C8 to L3 spinal segments
Ref. 7 - p. 269

136. THE POSTERIOR SPINOCEREBELLAR TRACT CONVEYS IMPULSES:
A. From stretch, touch and pressure receptors to the cerebellum
B. From pain and temperature receptors to the cerebellum
C. From receptors on the opposite side of the body to the cerebellum
D. From cells of Clarke's nucleus to the opposite cerebellar cortex
E. From cells of Clarke's nucleus to relay nuclei of thalamus
Ref. 7 - p. 272

137. THE ANTERIOR SPINOCEREBELLAR TRACT IS SITUATED__________IN THE SPINAL CORD:
A. In the anterior funiculus
B. Anterior to the spinotectal tract
C. Lateral to the lateral spino-thalamic tract
D. In the posterior funiculus
E. Lateral to the anterior corticospinal tract
Ref. 7 - p. 272

138. ALL OF THE STATEMENTS CONCERNING DISTRIBUTION OF THE ANTERIOR SPINOCEREBELLAR TRACT ARE TRUE, EXCEPT:
A. Neuron I is located in the dorsal root ganglion
B. Neuron II is located in the cell column at the base of the anterior and posterior horns in lumbar spinal segments
C. Fibers course along the dorsal surface of the superior cerebellar peduncle
D. Small number of fibers cross in the cerebellum
E. Fibers terminate primarily in the posterior lobe of the cerebellum
Ref. 7 - p. 272

139. THE ANTERIOR SPINOCEREBELLAR TRACT TRANSMITS IMPULSES:
A. From visceral receptors
B. From Meissner's corpuscles
C. Related to movement or posture of limb
D. Related to stretching of gut wall
E. Related to tension in individual muscles
Ref. 7 - p. 273

140. THE TRANSMISSION OF IMPULSES IN THE ANTERIOR SPINOCEREBELLAR TRACT IS NOT INFLUENCED BY THE:
A. Supraspinal system
B. Monosynaptic excitation from ipsilateral flexor reflex afferents
C. Monosynaptic excitation from contralateral flexor reflex afferents
D. Monosynaptic inhibition from ipsilateral and contralateral flexor reflex afferents
E. Polysynaptic excitation and inhibition from ipsilateral and contralateral extensor reflex afferents
Ref. 7 - p. 273

141. COMPONENTS OF THE CUNEOCEREBELLAR TRACT DO NOT INCLUDE:
A. Activation of Neuron I by touch and pressure receptors
B. The accessory cuneate nucleus
C. Afferent fibers via the dorsal roots from C1 to T7
D. Posterior external arcuate fibers
E. The contralateral cerebellar cortex
Ref. 7 - p. 273

142. THE SPINORETICULAR FIBERS TERMINATE ON CELLS OF THE FOLLOWING NUCLEI, EXCEPT THE:
A. Nucleus reticularis giganto cellularis on the same side
B. Lateral reticular on the same side
C. Reticularis giganto cellularis on the opposite side
D. Reticularis pontis on the same side
E. Reticularis pontis on the opposite side
Ref. 7 - p. 273

143. THE SPINORETICULAR FIBERS ORIGINATE FROM:
A. Upper cervical spinal segments and medulla primarily
B. All spinal levels
C. Spinal levels C8 to L3
D. The intermediomedial nucleus
E. The lateral reticular nucleus Ref. 7 - p. 273

144. ASCENDING FIBER SYSTEMS IN THE SPINAL CORD WHOSE FUNCTIONAL SIGNIFICANCE IS OBSCURED INCLUDE THE FOLLOWING, EXCEPT THE:
A. Spinocortical
B. Spino-olivary
C. Spinovestibular
D. Spinopontine
E. Anterior spinothalamic Ref. 7 - p. 274

145. LOCATED BETWEEN THE SPINOCEREBELLAR TRACT AND THE LATERAL FASCICULUS PROPRIUS AT THE LEVEL OF SPINAL SEGMENT C8 IS THE__________TRACT:
A. Spinotectal
B. Tectospinal
C. Lateral reticulospinal
D. Lateral spinothalamic
E. Lateral corticospinal Ref. 7 - p. 275

146. WHAT PERCENT OF FIBERS IN THE PYRAMIDAL TRACT CROSS IN THE PYRAMIDAL DECUSSATION?:
A. 40
B. 20
C. 60
D. 85
E. 100
Ref. 7 - p. 275

147. THE CORTICOSPINAL OR PYRAMIDAL TRACTS ORIGINATE FROM:
A. Purkinje cells
B. Area 44 of Brodmann
C. Frontal and temporal cortices
D. The precentral gyrus and adjacent cortical areas
E. The postcentral gyrus and adjacent cortical areas
Ref. 7 - p. 274

148. THE CORTICOSPINAL TRACT IS COMPOSED OF FIBERS:
A. Whose number exceeds one million in each tract
B. Which are predominantly (90%) 10 to 22 micra in diameter
C. The majority of which are unmyelinated
D. All of which decussate in the pyramid
E. All of which decussate in the anterior white commissure
Ref. 7 - p. 274

149. THE ANTERIOR OR DIRECT PYRAMIDAL TRACT IS LOCATED:
A. In the anterior funiculus of all spinal cord segments
B. Adjacent to the anterior median fissure of cervical and upper thoracic spinal segments
C. Just dorsal to the exit of the ventral root fibers
D. In the lateral funiculus anterior to the lateral pyramidal tract
E. In the anterior limb of the internal capsule
Ref. 7 - p. 275

150. CONCERNING FUNCTIONS OF THE PYRAMIDAL TRACT:
A. Is fully myelinated at birth
B. Controls primarily skilled volitional movements
C. Controls gross unskilled movements only
D. Is part of the extrapyramidal system controlling coordination of movement
E. Provides direct innervation of striated muscle by axons of Betz cells
Ref. 7 - p. 279

151. WHICH OF THE FOLLOWING CONSTITUTE THE UPPER MOTOR NEURONS?:
A. Anterior horn cells
B. Pyramidal cells
C. Renshaw cells
D. Betz cells
E. Oligodendrocytes
Ref. 7 - p. 279

152. IT HAS BEEN ESTIMATED THAT ABOUT________PERCENT OF ALL PYRAMIDAL FIBERS END IN THE CERVICAL CORD:
A. 25
B. 44
C. 85
D. 100
E. 55
Ref. 7 - p. 278

153. EXPERIMENTAL STUDIES HAVE DEMONSTRATED THAT STIMULATION OF THE BRAIN STEM RETICULAR FORMATION CAN EFFECT THE FOLLOWING FUNCTIONS, <u>EXCEPT</u>:
A. Facilitate or inhibit voluntary movement
B. Affect respiration
C. Exert pressor or depressor effect on the circulatory system
D. Exert depressant effects on the central transmission of sensory impulses
E. Facilitate peripheral transmission of sensory impulses
Ref. 7 - p. 280

154. THE RETICULOSPINAL TRACT ORIGINATES MAINLY FROM THE:
A. Small pyramidal cells of cerebral cortex
B. Basal nuclei
C. Thalamic nuclei
D. Nuclei of pontile and medullary reticular formation
E. Intermediolateral nucleus
Ref. 7 - p. 280

155. THE VESTIBULOSPINAL TRACT ORIGINATES FROM THE________ VESTIBULAR NUCLEUS:
A. Superior
B. Inferior
C. Medial
D. Lateral
E. None of the above
Ref. 7 - p. 282

156. THE VESTIBULOSPINAL TRACT DESCENDS:
A. Crossed in the anterior funiculus
B. Uncrossed in the lateral funiculus
C. Somatotopically organized
D. To the level of upper thoracic cord segments
E. The entire length of the spinal cord terminating on motor neurons of the ventral horns (central and anterolateral groups)
Ref. 7 - p. 282

157. THE VESTIBULOSPINAL TRACT RELAYS IMPULSES:
A. From cerebellar vermis and fastigial nuclei to the spinal cord
B. From medial vestibular nuclei to motor neurons on the opposite side
C. That are inhibitory to spinal mechanisms which control muscle tone
D. That are excitatory to flexor motor neurons
E. From sensory receptors in the organ of Corti to the motor neurons in the spinal cord Ref. 7 - p. 282

158. THE MOST IMPORTANT FUNCTION OF THE RUBROSPINAL TRACT IS:
A. Control of muscle tone in flexor muscle groups
B. Control of muscle tone in extensor muscle groups
C. Coordination of movement in the upper and lower extremities
D. Inhibition of visceral motor neurones in the spinal cord
E. Excitation of visceral motor neurones in the spinal cord
Ref. 7 - p. 287

159. THE VENTRAL TEGMENTAL DECUSSATION IS FORMED BY THE:
A. Tectospinal tract
B. Tectobulbar tract
C. Reticulospinal tract
D. Rubrospinal tract
E. Medial longitudinal fasciculus Ref. 7 - p. 285

160. IN MAN, THE RUBROSPINAL TRACT DOES NOT RELAY IMPULSES FROM THE:
A. Cerebellum to the spinal cord
B. Cerebral motor cortex to the spinal cord
C. Red nucleus to all levels of the spinal cord
D. Red nucleus to cervical and thoracic spinal cord segments
E. Red nucleus to cerebellum, facial nucleus and lateral reticular nucleus via collaterals Ref. 7 - p. 286

161. THE TECTOSPINAL TRACT EXTENDS FROM THE:
A. Red nucleus to the spinal cord
B. Pretectal area to the spinal cord segments
C. Superior colliculus to cervical spinal segments
D. Inferior colliculus to thoracic spinal segments
E. Inferior colliculus to all spinal segments
Ref. 7 - p. 287

162. THE DESCENDING FIBERS OF THE MEDIAL LONGITUDINAL FASCICULUS IN THE SPINAL CORD ORIGINATE FROM ALL THE STRUCTURES LISTED BELOW, <u>EXCEPT</u> THE:
A. Medial vestibular nucleus
B. Reticular formation
C. Superior colliculus
D. Interstitial nucleus of Cajal
E. Inferior colliculus Ref. 7 - p. 287

163. ASCENDING AND DESCENDING FIBERS WHICH BEGIN AND END IN THE SPINAL CORD AND CONNECT ITS VARIOUS LEVELS CONSTITUTE THE:
A. Fasciculus gracilis
B. Fasciculus cuneatus
C. Lateral reticulospinal tract
D. Medial longitudinal fasciculus
E. Fasciculus proprius Ref. 7 - p. 288

164. THE "FINAL COMMON PATHWAY" REFERS TO THE:
A. Purkinje cells and their axons
B. Betz cells and their axons
C. Pyramidal tract
D. Anterior horn cells and their axons
E. Dorsal root ganglion cells and their processes
Ref. 7 - p. 289

165. THE GRADUAL REPLACEMENT OF SPINAL FIBERS IN THE ZONE OF LISSAUER BY DESCENDING SPINAL TRIGEMINAL FIBERS OCCURS AT WHICH OF THE FOLLOWING AREAS?:
A. Thalamus
B. Hypothalamus
C. Pons
D. Midbrain
E. Medulla
Ref. 7 - p. 298

166. PHYLOGENETICALLY, ONE OF THE OLDEST PORTIONS OF THE NEURAXIS IS THE:
A. Reticular formation
B. Posterior funiculus
C. Corticospinal tract
D. Lateral spinothalamic tract
E. Ventral spinocerebellar tract Ref. 7 - p. 298

167. THE FIRST APPEARANCE OF THE NUCLEI OF THE POSTERIOR COLUMNS, AND THE DEVELOPMENT OF THE MEDULLARY RETICULAR FORMATION OCCURS AT WHICH OF THE FOLLOWING AREAS?:
A. Pons
B. Cervical spinal cord
C. Midbrain
D. Medulla
E. Diencephalon
Ref. 7 - p. 300

168. THE GREATLY ENLARGED SUBSTANTIA GELATINOSA IS CAPPED EXTERNALLY BY THE:
A. Ventral spinocerebellar pathway
B. Lateral spinothalamic tract
C. Tract of Lissauer
D. Lateral corticospinal tract
E. Dorsal spinocerebellar pathway Ref. 7 - p. 301

169. SPECIAL VISCERAL AFFERENT (SVA) FIBERS ARE COMPONENTS OF THE ________ CRANIAL NERVE:
A. Facial
B. Optic
C. Oculomotor
D. Trigeminal
E. Accessory Ref. 7 - p. 299

170. SPECIAL VISCERAL EFFERENT (SVE) FIBERS CONSTITUTE PART OF CRANIAL NERVE__________:
A. I
B. II
C. III
D. IV
E. V
Ref. 7 - p. 168

171. THE AUDITORY COMPONENT OF THE EIGHTH CRANIAL NERVE IS CLASSIFIED AS:
A. General somatic afferent (GSA)
B. General visceral afferent (GVA)
C. Special visceral afferent (SVA)
D. Special somatic afferent (SSA)
E. Special visceral efferent (SVE) Ref. 7 - p. 299

172. THE DORSAL ROOT FIBERS IN THE FASCICULUS GRACILIS TERMINATE:
A. On cells of nucleus gracilis of the opposite site
B. Somatotopically on cells of nucleus gracilis of the same side
C. In part in the inferior olivary nuclear complex
D. On cells of nucleus fastigii
E. None of the above Ref. 7 - p. 305

173. THE INTERNAL ARCUATE FIBERS ORIGINATE FROM CELLS OF THE:
A. Motor area of cerebral cortex
B. Cerebellar cortex
C. Dentate nucleus
D. Inferior olivary complex
E. Nucleus gracilis and cuneatus Ref. 7 - p. 307

174. THE FIBERS OF THE MEDIAL LEMNISCUS ORIGINATE FROM CELLS OF THE:
A. Cochlear nuclei
B. Vestibular nuclei
C. Inferior olivary complex
D. Trigeminal nuclei
E. Gracilis and cuneatus nuclei Ref. 7 - p. 307

175. CELLS OF THE ACCESSORY CUNEATE NUCLEUS GIVE RISE TO WHICH OF THE FOLLOWING?:
A. Crossed cuneocerebellar fibers
B. Uncrossed cuneocerebellar fibers
C. Fibers conveying impulses from receptors in muscles of the upper extremity
D. Fibers conveying pain and temperature to the thalamus
E. The medial lemniscus Ref. 7 - p. 311

176. FIBERS TERMINATING IN THE ACCESSORY CUNEATE NUCLEUS ARE DERIVED FROM:
A. Dorsal roots of all spinal nerves
B. Dorsal roots of cervical and upper thoracic segments
C. Dorsal roots distal to mid thoracic segments
D. Clarke's nucleus
E. Cells of lamina VI, VII and VIII Ref. 7 - p. 310

177. THE CELLS OF THE ACCESSORY CUNEATE NUCLEUS GIVE RISE TO FIBERS THAT:
A. Form the internal arcuate fibers
B. Terminate in the posterolateral nucleus of the thalamus
C. Contribute to the formation of lateral lemniscus
D. Contribute to the formation of medial lemniscus
E. Enter the cerebellum uncrossed via the inferior cerebellar peduncle
Ref. 7 - p. 311

178. THE SPINAL TRIGEMINAL TRACT EXTENDS FROM THE PONS TO:
A. Thalamus
B. Trapezoid body
C. Upper cervical segments
D. Lumbar segments
E. Entire length of the spinal cord Ref. 7 - p. 311

179. THE SPINAL TRIGEMINAL TRACT IS ORGANIZED SO THAT:
A. Fibers of the mandibular division are most ventral
B. Fibers of the opthalmic division are most ventral
C. Fibers of the maxillary division are most ventral
D. Fibers of the maxilla division are most dorsal
E. Fibers of the opthalmic division are most dorsal
Ref. 7 - p. 311

180. GENERAL SOMATIC AFFERENT FIBERS FROM THE__________NERVES CONTRIBUTE TO THE FORMATION OF THE SPINAL TRIGEMINAL TRACT:
A. Oculomotor
B. Trochlear
C. Abducens
D. Vagus
E. Accessory
Ref. 7 - p. 312

181. DESCENDING FIBERS IN THE SPINAL TRIGEMINAL TRACT CONVEY IMPULSES CONCERNED WITH:
A. Pain
B. Conscious proprioception
C. Temperature
D. Subconscious proprioception
E. All of the above Ref. 7 - p. 312

182. THE AREA POSTREMA CONTAINS WHICH OF THE FOLLOWING?:
A. Arterioles
B. Sinusoids
C. Purkinje cells
D. Amphicytes
E. Astroblast-like cells
Ref. 7 - p. 314

183. IMMEDIATELY ROSTRAL TO THE OBEX ON EACH SIDE OF THE FOURTH VENTRICLE IS A ROUNDED EMINENCE COMPOSED OF ASTROBLAST-LIKE CELLS, ARTERIOLES, SINUSOIDS, AND APOLAR AND UNIPOLAR NEURONS. IT IS RECOGNIZED AS THE:
A. Dorsal motor nucleus of vagus
B. Nucleus of fasciculus solitarius
C. Area postrema
D. Paramedian reticular nucleus
E. Arcuate nucleus Ref. 7 - p. 314

184. THE LATERAL RETICULAR NUCLEUS IS LOCATED:
A. Dorsal to inferior olive and ventral to spinal trigeminal nucleus
B. Dorsal to spinal trigeminal nucleus
C. Ventral to inferior olivary nucleus
D. Lateral to hypoglossal nucleus
E. Between nucleus ambiguus and nucleus reticularis gigantocellularis
Ref. 7 - p. 314

185. AFFERENT FIBERS TO THE ARCUATE NUCLEUS ARE DERIVED FROM THE CEREBRAL CORTEX, AND EFFERENT FIBERS PROJECT:
A. Uncrossed to cervical spinal cord segments
B. Crossed as arcuate fibers to the cerebellum
C. Uncrossed to cerebellum
D. Crossed to cervical spinal cord segments
E. Uncrossed to cervical and thoracic spinal cord segments
Ref. 7 - p. 314

186. THE FLOOR OF THE FOURTH VENTRICLE CONTAINS THREE EMINENCES ARRANGED IN THE FOLLOWING ORDER FROM MEDIAL TO LATERAL:
A. Trigonum hypoglossi, trigonum vagi, and area vestibularis
B. Trigonum hypoglossi, area vestibularis, and trigonum vagi
C. Trigonum vagi, trigonum hypoglossi, and area vestibularis
D. Pyramid, trigonum hypoglossi and area vestibularis
Ref. 7 - p. 315

187. AXONS OF CELLS FORMING THE INFERIOR OLIVARY COMPLEX TERMINATE IN THE:
A. Ventral lateral nucleus of the thalamus
B. Posterolateral nucleus of the thalamus
C. Spinal cord of the opposite side
D. Spinal cord on the same side
E. Cerebellum of the opposite side Ref. 7 - p. 316

188. THE TERM AMICULUM OLIVAE REFERS TO:
A. A surface elevation on the medulla in the area of the olivary nuclei
B. Axons of cells in the olivary nucleus forming a fiber bundle which enters the cerebellum
C. Descending fibers terminating upon cells of the inferior olive arising from cerebral cortex, red nucleus and periaqueductal gray
D. Descending fibers from the hypothalamus terminating in the inferior olivary complex
E. Axons of cells of cerebellar nuclei terminating in the inferior olivary complex Ref. 7 - p. 316

189. CONCERNING THE MEDULLARY RETICULAR FORMATION, IT IS:
A. Formed entirely by a multineuronal sensory chain terminating in the thalamus
B. Formed by a multineuronal chain conveying motor impulses to the spinal cord only
C. Phylogenetically the newest addition to the CNS
D. Phylogenetically very old
E. A diffuse mass of nuclei and fibers with no recognizable functions
Ref. 7 - p. 316

190. FIBERS FORMING THE INFERIOR CEREBELLAR PEDUNCLE DO NOT INCLUDE THE:
A. Posterior spinocerebellar tract
B. Olivocerebellar fibers
C. Pontocerebellar fibers
D. Axons of cells in the arcuate nucleus
E. Fibers of the lateral reticular nucleus of the medulla
Ref. 7 - p. 188

191. THE HYPOGLOSSAL NERVE IS FORMED BY FIBERS WHICH:
A. Emerge from the ventrolateral sulcus of upper four cervical nerves
B. Conduct special visceral efferent fibers
C. Innervate the genioglossus muscle
D. Originate from cells that occupy the central gray of the median eminence
E. Innervate the masticatory muscles Ref. 7 - p. 319

192. WHICH OF THE FOLLOWING NUCLEAR MASSES CONSTITUTE THE SO-CALLED PERIHYPOGLOSSAL NUCLEI?:
A. Dorsal motor nucleus
B. Nucleus intercalatus
C. Nucleus prepositus
D. Nucleus of Roller
E. Nucleus ambiguus
Ref. 7 - p. 320

193. THE CRANIAL ROOT OF THE ACCESSORY NERVE ARISES FROM NEURONS IN THE:
A. Anterior horn cells C1-3
B. Dorsal motor nucleus of vagus
C. Nucleus ambiguus
D. Salivatory nucleus
E. Nucleus solitarius Ref. 7 - p. 320

194. THE CRANIAL FIBERS OF THE ACCESSORY NERVE JOIN THE VAGUS AND INNERVATE THE:
A. Sternomastoid muscle
B. Trapezius muscle
C. Masticatory muscles
D. Cricothyroid muscle
E. Intrinsic muscles of the larynx Ref. 7 - p. 320

195. THE ROOTLETS OF THE SPINAL PART OF THE ACCESSORY NERVE UNITE TO FORM A COMMON TRUNK (EXTERNAL BRANCH) WHICH EXITS FROM THE SPINAL CANAL THROUGH FORAMEN:
A. Intervertebrale
B. Magnum
C. Ovale
D. Spinosum
E. Jugulare
Ref. 7 - p. 321

196. FIBERS WHICH FORM THE VAGUS NERVE DO NOT INCLUDE:
A. General visceral efferent fibers
B. Special visceral efferent fibers
C. General somatic efferent fibers
D. General somatic afferent fibers
E. General visceral afferent fibers Ref. 7 - p. 321

197. THE GENERAL SOMATIC AFFERENT FIBERS OF THE VAGUS NERVE SUPPLYING THE SKIN IN BACK OF THE EAR HAVE THEIR CELL BODIES IN THE__________GANGLION:
A. Dorsal root of C_{1-5}
B. Trigeminal
C. Superior of vagus nerve
D. Inferior of vagus nerve
E. Dorsal root of C_2 Ref. 7 - p. 321

198. THE SPECIAL VISCERAL EFFERENT FIBERS OF THE VAGUS NERVE INNERVATE:
A. Smooth muscle of the gastrointestinal tract
B. Secretory glands of the intestinal mucosa
C. Striated muscles of the larynx and pharynx
D. Cardiac muscle
E. Taste receptors at the root of the tongue
Ref. 7 - p. 322

199. THE FOLLOWING FIBERS TERMINATE IN THE NUCLEUS AMBIGUUS, EXCEPT THE:
A. Corticobulbar
B. Secondary vagal
C. Secondary glossopharyngeal
D. Secondary trigeminal
E. Secondary hypoglossal Ref. 7 - p. 322

200. CUTANEOUS FIBERS CONTAINED IN THE AURICULAR BRANCH OF THE VAGUS NERVE TERMINATE IN THE__________NUCLEUS:
A. Ambiguus
B. Solitary
C. Dorsal motor
D. Main sensory trigeminal
E. Spinal trigeminal
Ref. 7 - p. 322

201. THE FASICULUS SOLITARIUS IS FORMED BY FIBERS CONTRIBUTED BY THE:
A. Accessory nerve
B. Trigeminal nerve
C. Vagus, glossopharyngeal and facial nerves
D. Medullary reticular nuclei
E. Tectum Ref. 7 - p. 323

202. SPECIAL VISCERAL AFFERENT FIBERS (TASTE) FROM IX AND VII CRANIAL NERVES TERMINATE MAINLY IN THE:
A. Rostral end of nucleus solitarius (gustatory nucleus)
B. Caudal end of nucleus solitarius
C. Nucleus ambiguus
D. Main sensory trigeminal nucleus
E. Spinal trigeminal nucleus Ref. 7 - p. 324

203. THE CAUDAL PART OF THE MEDIAL NUCLEUS SOLITARIUS PROJECTS TO DORSAL AND LATERAL RETICULAR FORMATION OF THE MEDULLA WHICH REGULATE ALL THE LISTED FUNCTIONS, EXCEPT:
A. Respiratory
B. Cardiovascular
C. Emetic
D. Laryngeal reflex Ref. 7 - p. 324

204. THE "RESPIRATORY CENTER" CONCERNED WITH MAINTENANCE OF RESPIRATORY MOVEMENTS IS LOCATED IN THE:
A. Tegmentum of metencephalon
B. Tectum of mesencephalon
C. Reticular formation of medulla
D. Thalamus
E. Upper cervical spinal segments Ref. 7 - p. 324

205. THE ROSTRAL ENLARGED PORTION OF THE NUCLEUS SOLITARIUS, WHICH RECEIVED SPECIAL VISCERAL AFFERENT FIBERS MAINLY FROM THE FACIAL AND GLOSSOPHARYNGEAL NERVES, IS REFERRED TO AS THE:
A. Nucleus ambiguus
B. Gustatory nucleus
C. Inferior salivatory nucleus
D. Dorsal longitudinal fasciculus
E. Nucleus intercalatus Ref. 7 - p. 324

206. FUNCTIONAL COMPONENTS OF THE GLOSSOPHARYNGEAL NERVE INCLUDE THE FOLLOWING FIBERS, EXCEPT:
A. General somatic afferent
B. General somatic efferent
C. General visceral afferent
D. General visceral efferent
E. Special visceral efferent Ref. 7 - p. 325

207. THE REFLEX SLOWING OF THE HEART RATE AND FALL IN THE BLOOD PRESSURE INVOLVES THE FOLLOWING STRUCTURES, EXCEPT THE:
A. Carotid sinus
B. Carotid sinus nerve (N. IX)
C. Superior salivatory nucleus
D. Dorsal motor nucleus of X
E. Parasympathetic fibers (N. X) to sinoatrial and atrioventricular node
Ref. 7 - p. 325

208. INNERVATION OF THE PAROTID GLAND INVOLVES THE FOLLOWING NEURAL STRUCTURES, EXCEPT THE:
A. Dorsal motor nucleus of the vagus
B. Inferior salivatory nucleus
C. General visceral efferent fibers
D. Lesser petrosal nerve
E. Otic ganglion Ref. 7 - p. 326

209. THE CORTICOBULBAR FIBERS FROM THE PRECENTRAL AND POSTCENTRAL GYRI ARE DISTRIBUTED TO ALL THE NUCLEI LISTED BELOW, EXCEPT:
A. Sensory relay nuclei
B. Parts of reticular formation
C. Certain motor cranial nerve nuclei
D. Basal ganglia Ref. 7 - p. 327

210. SENSORY RELAY NUCLEI RECEIVING CORTICOBULBAR FIBERS DO NOT INCLUDE THE:
A. Gracilis nucleus
B. Cuneatus nucleus
C. Sensory trigeminal nucleus
D. Nucleus of the solitary fasciculus
E. Thalamus

Ref. 7 - p. 327

211. CORTICORETICULAR FIBERS TERMINATE PRIMARILY IN WHICH OF THE FOLLOWING AREAS?:
A. Hippocampus
B. Hypothalamus
C. Pons
D. Medulla
E. Midbrain

Ref. 7 - p. 327

212. AT THE TRANSVERSE LEVEL OF THE LATERAL RECESS OF THE FOURTH VENTRICLE THE FOLLOWING NUCLEI ARE PRESENT:
A. Hypoglossal and dorsal motor nucleus of the vagus
B. Motor nucleus of the trigeminal
C. Oculomotor nucleus
D. Trochlear nucleus
E. Facial nucleus

Ref. 7 - p. 330

213. THE DORSAL COCHLEAR NUCLEUS FORMS A PROMINENCE IN THE RHOMBOID FOSSA KNOWN AS THE:
A. Medial eminence
B. Inferior colliculus
C. Tuberculum cuneatus
D. Tuberculum gracilis
E. Tuberculum acousticum

Ref. 7 - p. 331

214. ALL OF THE FOLLOWING CRANIAL NERVES ARE PRESENT AT THE JUNCTION OF THE MEDULLA AND PONS, EXCEPT THE:
A. Cochlear
B. Vestibular
C. Facial
D. Abducens
E. Trigeminal

Ref. 7 - p. 333

215. THE BASILAR PORTION OF THE PONS PROPER CONTAINS THE:
A. Tectospinal tract
B. Olivospinal tract
C. Rubrospinal tract
D. Corticospinal tract
E. Medial lemniscus

Ref. 7 - p. 335

216. THE MIDDLE CEREBELLAR PEDUNCLE CONTAINS__________FIBERS:
A. Spinocerebellar
B. Reticulocerebellar
C. Tectocerebellar
D. Pontocerebellar
E. Olivocerebellar

Ref. 7 - p. 336

217. THE PONTINE TEGMENTUM CONTAINS THE FOLLOWING CRANIAL NUCLEI, EXCEPT THE:
A. Vestibular
B. Cochlear
C. Facial
D. Trigeminal
E. Abducens

Ref. 7 - p. 338

218. ALL OF THE FOLLOWING STRUCTURES ARE PART OF THE PONTINE TEGMENTUM, EXCEPT THE:
A. Red nucleus
B. Trapezoid body
C. Spinal trigeminal nucleus and tract
D. Vestibular nuclei
E. Nucleus of the medial eminence Ref. 7 - p. 338

219. THE ROOT FIBERS OF THE MOTOR NUCLEUS OF N. VII FOLLOW THE FOLLOWING ROUTE, EXCEPT:
A. Emerging from the nucleus proceed dorsomedially
B. Ascend for 2 mm. medial to the abducens nucleus
C. Ascend dorsal to the medial longitudinal fasciculus
D. Form the internal genu of the facial nerve
E. Pass ventromedially emerging at midline at the pontomedullary junction Ref. 7 - p. 340

220. WHICH OF THE FOLLOWING STRUCTURES IS NOT INVOLVED IN CONDUCTION OF AUDITORY IMPULSES?:
A. Organ of Corti
B. Spiral ganglion
C. Dorsal cochlear nucleus
D. Ventral cochlear nucleus
E. Superior colliculus Ref. 7 - p. 341

221. THE DORSAL AND VENTRAL COCHLEAR NUCLEI ARE LOCATED:
A. Dorsolateral to inferior cerebellar peduncle
B. Ventromedial to inferior cerebellar peduncle
C. In pontine tegmentum
D. Lateral to brachium conjunctivum
E. Medial to vestibular nuclei Ref. 7 - p. 341

222. WHICH OF THE FOLLOWING STATEMENTS CONCERNING TONOTOPIC LOCALIZATION IN THE AUDITORY SYSTEM IS INCORRECT?:
A. High tones are received in the basal coils of cochlea
B. Low frequencies are received in the apical portion of cochlea
C. Apical cochlear fibers terminate in ventral part of dorsal cochlear nucleus
D. Basal cochlear fibers end in the dorsal cochlear nucleus and in the ventral nucleus
E. Apical cochlear fibers and basal cochlear fibers end in ventral cochlear nucleus Ref. 7 - p. 342

223. WHICH OF THE FOLLOWING STATEMENTS CONCERNING THE SECONDARY AUDITORY PATHWAYS IS INCORRECT?:
A. The ventral acoustic stria participate in the formation of the trapezoid body
B. Fibers of ventral acoustic stria form in part the lateral lemniscus
C. The ventral acoustic striae arise from the ventral cochlear nucleus
D. The dorsal stria crosses the median raphe and joins the lateral lemniscus
E. Fibers from the cochlear nuclei ascend in the ipsilateral lemniscus
Ref. 7 - p. 345

224. ALL OF THE FOLLOWING NEURONES ARE INVOLVED IN THE AUDITORY PATHWAY, EXCEPT THE:
A. Cells of the spiral ganglion
B. Cells of the dorsal and ventral cochlear nuclei
C. Nuclei of the superior olivary complex
D. Nucleus of the lateral lemniscus
E. Cells of the superior colliculus Ref. 7 - p. 346

225. THE AUDITORY RADIATION PROJECTS TO THE:
A. Postcentral gyrus
B. Precentral gyrus
C. Superior frontal gyrus
D. Transverse temporal gyrus of Heschl
E. Cingulate gyrus Ref. 7 - p. 346

226. THE MEDIAL GENICULATE BODY GIVES RISE TO GENICULOCORTICAL FIBERS WHICH PROJECT TO WHICH OF THE FOLLOWING AREAS?:
A. Parahippocampal gyri
B. Parietal cortex
C. Post-central gyri
D. Pre-central gyri
E. Transverse temporal gyri of Heschl Ref. 7 - p. 347

227. DIFFUSE CELLULAR AGGREGATIONS INTERPOSED IN THE COURSE OF THE LATERAL LEMNISCUS IN THE UPPER PORTION OF THE PONS INCLUDE WHICH OF THE FOLLOWING?:
A. Superior olive
B. Nucleus of the lateral lemniscus
C. Restiform body
D. Nucleus of the abducens
E. Ventral cochlear nucleus Ref. 7 - p. 345

228. THE VESTIBULAR PORTION OF THE INNER EAR CONSISTS OF:
A. Semicircular canals
B. Utricle
C. Saccule
D. Trapezoid body
E. Acoustic tubercle Ref. 7 - p. 347

229. ALL OF THE FOLLOWING STRUCTURES ARE ASSOCIATED WITH EQUILIBRIUM AND ORIENTATION IN SPACE, EXCEPT THE:
A. Crista ampullaris
B. Organ of Corti
C. Macula utriculi
D. Macula sacculi
E. Otoliths Ref. 7 - p. 347

230. VESTIBULAR ROOT FIBERS TERMINATE IN THE:
A. Cortex of the nodulus, uvula and flocculus
B. Inferior colliculus
C. Superior olivary nuclei
D. Nucleus of the lateral lemniscus
E. Nucleus of the trapezoid body Ref. 7 - p. 348

231. UPON ENTERING THE BRAIN STEM, PRIMARY VESTIBULAR FIBERS BIFURCATE AND TERMINATE IN THE FOLLOWING ORDER:
A. Ascending fibers terminate in the superior vestibular nucleus only
B. Ascending fibers terminate in the superior, medial and lateral vestibular nuclei
C. Ascending fibers terminate in the medial vestibular nucleus only
D. Descending fibers terminate in the lateral vestibular nucleus only
E. Descending fibers terminate in medial and lateral vestibular nuclei
Ref. 7 - p. 350

232. THE EFFERENT CEREBELLAR FIBERS PLUS BOTH PRIMARY AND SECONDARY VESTIBULOCEREBELLAR FIBERS FORM THE:
A. Internal arcuate fibers
B. External arcuate fibers
C. Brachium pontis
D. Juxtarestiform body
E. Brachium conjunctivum
Ref. 7 - p. 351

233. THE VESTIBULAR NUCLEI GIVE RISE TO SECONDARY VESTIBULAR FIBERS WHICH PROJECT TO THE:
A. Inferior olive
B. Cerebral cortex
C. Cerebellar cortex
D. Dentate nucleus
E. Red nucleus
Ref. 7 - p. 351

234. THE DESCENDING VESTIBULAR FIBERS IN THE MEDIAL LONGITUDINAL FASCICULUS PROJECTING TO SPINAL LEVELS ARISE PRIMARILY IN:
A. Superior vestibular nucleus
B. Medial vestibular nucleus
C. Lateral vestibular nucleus
D. Inferior vestibular nucleus
E. All vestibular nuclei
Ref. 7 - p. 353

235. THE DESCENDING VESTIBULAR FIBERS IN THE MEDIAL LONGITUDINAL FASCICULUS PROJECT:
A. Crossed fibers only
B. The whole length of the spinal cord
C. To the lower thoracic spinal segments
D. To the cervical spinal segments
E. To the lumbar spinal segments
Ref. 7 - p. 353

236. ALL OF THE FOLLOWING NONVESTIBULAR DESCENDING FIBERS CONTRIBUTE TO THE FORMATION OF MEDIAL LONGITUDINAL FASCICULUS, EXCEPT THE:
A. Interstitiospinal tract
B. Tectobulbar and tectospinal
C. Reticulospinal
D. Corticospinal
Ref. 7 - p. 353

237. THE ASCENDING VESTIBULAR FIBERS IN THE MEDIAL LONGITUDINAL FASCICULUS PROJECT TO THE FOLLOWING AREAS, WITH THE EXCEPTION OF THE:
A. Abducens nucleus
B. Trochlear nucleus
C. Oculomotor nucleus
D. Interstitial nucleus of Cajal
E. Postcentral gyrus Ref. 7 - p. 354

238. THE SECONDARY VESTIBULAR FIBERS CONTAINED IN THE MEDIAL LONGITUDINAL FASCICULUS ARE ESSENTIAL FOR:
A. Pupillary reflex
B. Conjugate eye movements
C. Corneal reflex
D. Closing of eyes due to loud noise
E. Lacrimal reflex Ref. 7 - p. 356

239. ALL OF THE LISTED FIBER TRACTS ARE AFFERENT TO THE FACIAL MOTOR NUCLEUS, EXCEPT THE:
A. Trigeminal fibers
B. Direct corticobulbar fibers
C. Indirect corticobulbar fibers
D. Crossed rubrobulbar fibers
E. Crossed spinal fibers Ref. 7 - p. 357

240. TASTE IMPULSES FROM THE ANTERIOR TWO-THIRDS OF THE TONGUE REACH THE:
A. Upper portion of the solitary nucleus
B. Lower portion of the solitary nucleus
C. Superior salivatory nucleus
D. Dorsal motor nucleus of X
E. Nucleus ambiguus Ref. 7 - p. 358

241. CONJUGATE LATERAL MOVEMENTS OF THE EYES ARE NOT FULLY UNDERSTOOD, BUT IT IS GENERALLY AGREED THAT FIBERS IN THE MEDIAL LONGITUDINAL FASCICULUS INTERCONNECT WHICH OF THE FOLLOWING ESSENTIAL NUCLEI?:
A. Abducens
B. Facial
C. Trochlear
D. Hypoglossal
E. Oculomotor
Ref. 7 - p. 360

242. SPECIAL VISCERAL EFFERENT FIBERS OF THE TRIGEMINAL NERVE INNERVATE WHICH OF THE FOLLOWING?:
A. Muscles of mastication
B. Tensor tympani
C. Levator veli palatini
D. Zygomatic masar
E. Tensor veli palatini Ref. 7 - p. 364

243. ALL OF THE STRUCTURES LISTED BELOW ARE LOCATED IN A TRANSVERSE SECTION THROUGH THE PONS AT THE LEVEL OF ROOT FIBERS OF THE TRIGEMINAL NERVE, EXCEPT THE:
A. Central tegmental tract
B. Nucleus reticularis pontis oralis
C. Nucleus sensorius principalis of V
D. Motor nucleus of V
E. Mesencephalic nucleus of V Ref. 7 - p. 363

244. THE TRIGEMINAL NERVE CONVEYS TOUCH, PAIN, AND THERMAL SENSE FROM ALL THE LISTED REGIONS OF THE BODY, EXCEPT:
A. The skin of the face and forehead
B. The skin of the occipital area of the scalp and most of the external ear
C. The ectodermal mucous membranes of the nose, the nasal sinuses and the oral cavity
D. The teeth
E. Most of the cranial dura Ref. 7 - p. 364

245. PROPRIOCEPTIVE IMPULSES ARE CONVEYED BY THE TRIGEMINAL NERVE FROM ALL LISTED STRUCTURES, WITH THE EXCEPTION OF THE:
A. Teeth
B. Hard palate
C. Temporomandibular joint
D. Muscles of mastication
E. Suprahyoid muscles Ref. 7 - p. 364

246. AFFERENT FIBERS OF THE MESENCEPHALIC NUCLEUS OF THE TRIGEMINAL NERVE CONVEY PROPRIOCEPTIVE IMPULSES FROM WHICH OF THE FOLLOWING?:
A. Levator angulii oris
B. Depressor labii inferioris
C. Hard palate
D. Peridontium
E. Muscles of mastication Ref. 7 - p. 368

247. THE NEURONS OF THE MESENCEPHALIC NUCLEUS OF N. V HAVE THE FOLLOWING CHARACTERISTIC FEATURES:
A. Large multipolar cells
B. Unipolar cells
C. Small multipolar cells
D. Multipolar cells with large vesicular nuclei and eccentric nucleolus Ref. 7 - p. 365

248. THE FIBERS CONSTITUTING THE DORSAL TRIGEMINAL TRACT REPRESENT:
A. Crossed secondary trigeminal fibers originating from the principal sensory nucleus of N. V
B. Crossed secondary trigeminal fibers originating from the spinal nucleus of N. V
C. Crossed secondary trigeminal fibers originating from the mesencephalic nucleus of N. V
D. Uncrossed secondary trigeminal fibers originating in the principal sensory nucleus of N. V
E. Uncrossed secondary trigeminal fibers originating in the spinal spinal nucleus of N. V Ref. 7 - p. 371

249. ALL OF THE STATEMENTS BELOW CONCERNING THE VENTRAL TRIGEMINAL TRACT ARE CORRECT, EXCEPT THAT:
A. It is formed by axons originating in the spinal trigeminal nucleus
B. Fibers forming the tract originate in contralateral trigeminal nuclei
C. Fibers of this tract ascend with the contralateral medial lemniscus
D. Fibers of this tract, for the most part, terminate in the ventral posteromedial nucleus of the thalamus
E. Fibers of this tract descend contralaterally as spinal trigeminal tract
Ref. 7 - p. 370

250. SECONDARY REFLEX FIBERS ARISING FROM THE TERMINAL NUCLEI OF N. V TERMINATE AT ALL THE LISTED NUCLEI, EXCEPT:
A. The corneal reflex, to the motor nucleus of N. VII
B. The lacrimal or tearing reflex to the dorsal motor nucleus of N. X
C. Sneezing to the nucleus of N. XII, the nucleus ambiguus, phrenic and other respiratory nuclei
D. Salivary reflexes, to the salivatory nuclei of Nn. VII and IX
E. Oculocardiac reflex to the dorsal motor nucleus of N. X
Ref. 7 - p. 372

251. THE CHARACTERISTIC FEATURES OF THE ISTHMUS RHOMBENCEPHALI DO NOT INCLUDE THE:
A. Superior medullary velum
B. Cerebral aqueduct
C. Root fibers of trochlear nerve
D. Superior cerebellar peduncle
E. Superior olive Ref. 7 - p. 372

252. FIBERS FORMING THE SUPERIOR CEREBELLAR PEDUNCLE ORIGINATE FROM THE:
A. Anterior lobe of cerebellum
B. Posterior lobe of cerebellum
C. Flocculonodular lobe
D. Dentate, emboliform and globose nuclei
E. Red nucleus Ref. 7 - p. 373

253. ALL OF THE FOLLOWING STRUCTURES ARE FOUND IN THE SECTION OF THE MIDBRAIN AT THE LEVEL OF THE INFERIOR COLLICULUS, WITH THE EXCEPTION OF THE:
A. Cerebral aqueduct
B. Decussation of the cerebellar peduncles
C. Crura cerebri
D. Substantia nigra
E. Oculomotor nucleus Ref. 7 - p. 376

254. ALL STATEMENTS BELOW CONCERNING THE TROCHLEAR NERVE ARE TRUE, EXCEPT THAT:
A. The nucleus of the trochlear nerve is located at the level of the inferior colliculus just dorsal to medial longitudinal fasciculus
B. The intracranial root fibers originate and exit on the same side just inferior and lateral to the inferior colliculus
C. The nerve passes between the superior cerebellar and posterior cerebral arteries
D. Innervates the superior oblique muscle.
E. Lesion of the nerve produces diplopia which is vertical and maximal on attempted downward gaze to the opposite side
Ref. 7 - p. 377

255. ALL OF THE FOLLOWING STATEMENTS CONCERNING CONNECTIONS (AFFERENT AND EFFERENT) OF THE INFERIOR COLLICULUS ARE TRUE, EXCEPT:
A. Receives afferent fibers from the lateral lemniscus
B. Receives afferent fibers from the colliculus of the opposite side
C. Receives afferent fibers from the medial geniculate body
D. Efferent fibers project largely to the medial geniculate body
E. Efferent fibers project to the posterolateral nucleus of the thalamus
Ref. 7 - p. 378

256. ALL OF THE FOLLOWING STATEMENTS CONCERNING CONNECTIONS OF THE DORSAL TEGMENTAL NUCLEUS ARE TRUE, EXCEPT:
A. Receives fibers from the interpeduncular nucleus
B. Receives fibers from the mammillary bodies
C. Is related to dorsal longitudinal fasciculus
D. Gives origin to the tectospinal tract Ref. 7 - p. 379

257. ALL OF THE LISTED STRUCTURES ARE FOUND IN THE TRANSVERSE SECTION OF MIDBRAIN THROUGH THE SUPERIOR COLLICULUS, WITH THE EXCEPTION OF:
A. Oculomotor nuclei
B. Trochlear nuclei
C. Red nuclei
D. Brachium of the inferior colliculus
E. Central tegmental tract Ref. 7 - p. 380

258. AFFERENT CONNECTIONS OF THE SUPERIOR COLLICULUS DO NOT INCLUDE:
A. Fibers from the pallium
B. Fibers from the lateral geniculate body
C. Fibers from the retina
D. Spinotectal fibers
E. Fibers originating in cerebellar cortex
Ref. 7 - p. 382

259. EFFERENT FIBERS FROM THE SUPERIOR COLLICULUS DO NOT INCLUDE:
A. Tectoreticular fibers
B. Tectospinal tract
C. Tectopontine fibers
D. Brachium of the superior colliculus Ref. 7 - p. 382

260. ALL OF THE LISTED FIBERS FORM THE POSTERIOR COMMISSURE, EXCEPT:
A. Fibers from the habenular nuclei
B. Fibers from the prectectal nuclei
C. Fibers from the nucleus of the posterior commissure
D. Commissural fibers from the superior colliculi
E. Fibers from the interstitial nucleus Ref. 7 - p. 384

261. CHARACTERISTICS OF THE SUBCOMMISSURAL ORGAN DO NOT INCLUDE:
A. Location beneath the posterior commissure in the roof of the cerebral aqueduct
B. Secretory function
C. Serves as volume receptor
D. Only neurosecretory structure in the midbrain
E. Secretes thyrotropic hormones Ref. 7 - p. 384

262. THE GENERAL SOMATIC EFFERENT NUCLEI OF N. III ARE THE:
A. Lateral nuclear groups and caudal central nucleus
B. Anterior median nucleus
C. Nucleus of Edinger-Westphal
D. Nucleus of Perlia
E. Nucleus of Darkschewitsch Ref. 7 - p. 385

263. FIBERS FROM THE SUPERIOR COLLICULUS APPEAR TO REACH THE OCULOMOTOR NUCLEI VIA WHICH OF THE FOLLOWING?:
A. Medial longitudinal fasciculus
B. Interstitial nucleus of Cajal
C. Dorsal longitudinal fasciculus
D. Nucleus of Darkschewitsch
E. Brachium of the superior colliculus Ref. 7 - p. 388

264. THE PATHWAY FOR THE PUPILLARY LIGHT REFLEX DOES NOT INVOLVE:
A. Retina and axons of ganglion cells
B. Brachium of the superior colliculus
C. Cells of the superior colliculus
D. Axons of pretectal cells
E. Edinger-Westphal nucleus Ref. 7 - p. 389

265. THE ACCOMMODATION-CONVERGENCE REACTION DOES NOT INVOLVE:
A. Contraction of the medial recti muscles
B. Relaxation of ciliary muscle
C. Pupillary constriction
D. Visual cortex
E. Convergence center of N. III Ref. 7 - p. 389

266. EFFERENT PROJECTIONS OF THE RED NUCLEUS DO NOT INCLUDE __________ FIBERS:
A. Rubrotectal
B. Rubrocerebellar
C. Rubrobulbar
D. Rubrospinal
E. Rubro-olivary Ref. 7 - p. 391

267. WHICH OF THE RETICULAR NUCLEI IS NOT PART OF THE MESENCEPHALON?:
A. Nucleus tegmenti pedunculopontinus
B. Nucleus cuneiformis
C. Nucleus subcuneiformis
D. Nucleus reticularis gigantocellularis
Ref. 7 - p. 394

268. WHICH NUCLEI BELOW ARE NOT INCLUDED AMONG THE MESENCEPHALIC TEGMENTAL NUCLEI?:
A. Interstitial nuclei of Cajal
B. Nuclei of Darkschewitsch
C. Nuclei of the posterior commissure
D. Dorsal tegmental nuclei
E. Nuclei prepositi
Ref. 7 - p. 394

269. CHARACTERISTICS OF SUBSTANTIA NIGRA DO NOT INCLUDE:
A. Is the most voluminous nuclear mass of the mesencephalon
B. Large cells store a primary catecholamine (dopamine)
C. Parkinsonism (paralysis agitans) may by related to pathological condition of this nucleus
D. It is considered as an extrapyramidal nucleus
E. The nigro-spinal fibers project to lower thoracic spinal segments
Ref. 7 - p. 401

270. THE POSITION OF THE CORTICOPONTINE FIBERS IN THE CRUS CEREBRI IS:
A. Extreme medial and lateral portions
B. Most lateral of the central region
C. Middle region
D. Most medial of the central region
E. Lateral half
Ref. 7 - p. 404

271. THE PALEOCEREBELLUM IS FREQUENTLY REFERRED TO AS THE:
A. Flocculonodular lobe
B. Superior and inferior semilunar lobules
C. Uvula and tonsil
D. Anterior lobe
E. Posterior lobe
Ref. 7 - p. 405

272. THE CEREBELLAR CORTEX CONSISTS OF THE FOLLOWING LAYERS, WITH THE EXCEPTION OF THE:
A. Molecular layer
B. Granular layer
C. Purkinje cell layer
D. Multiform layer
Ref. 7 - p. 407

273. THE DENDRITIC RAMIFICATIONS OF THE BASKET CELLS ARE CONFINED TO THE __________ LAYER OF CEREBELLAR CORTEX:
A. Molecular layer
B. Purkinje cell layer
C. Outer part of granular layer
D. Middle part of granular layer
E. Inner part of the granular layer
Ref. 7 - p. 407

274. CHARACTERISTICS OF PURKINJE CELLS DO NOT INCLUDE:
A. Flask-shaped cell body
B. Dendritic tree which arborizes in a plane corresponding with the long axis of the folium
C. Terminal dendritic arborizations have short thick spines "gemmules"
D. Most axons pass to deep cerebellar nuclei
E. Axons are the only ones from the cortical neurones to enter the white matter
Ref. 7 - p. 408

275. WHICH OF THE FOLLOWING STATEMENTS CONCERNING MOSSY FIBERS IS INCORRECT?:
A. Pass into granular layer
B. Lose myelin sheath and give off many collaterals
C. Lobulated enlargements (rosettes occur along the course of the branches)
D. The rosettes form the center of each cerebellar glomerulus
E. Synapse with cell bodies of Purkinje cells
Ref. 7 - p. 412

276. AFFERENT FIBERS TO THE CEREBELLUM DO NOT INCLUDE THE:
A. Vestibulocerebellar fibers
B. Cochleocerebellar fibers
C. Posterior spinocerebellar tract
D. Anterior spinocerebellar tract
E. Cuneocerebellar fibers
Ref. 7 - p. 420

277. CEREBELLAR EFFERENT FIBERS ORIGINATING FROM THE FASTIGIAL NUCLEI EMERGE FROM THE CEREBELLUM VIA THE:
A. Superior cerebellar peduncle
B. Middle cerebellar peduncle
C. Inferior cerebellar peduncle
D. Uncinate fasciculus and the juxtarestiform body
Ref. 7 - p. 427

278. ALL OF THE FOLLOWING STATEMENTS ARE TRUE CONCERNING CEREBELLAR FUNCTION, EXCEPT:
A. Coordination of somatic motor activity
B. Regulation of muscle tone
C. Maintenance of equilibrium
D. Conscious appreciation of muscle, joint and tendon sense
Ref. 7 - p. 433

279. WHICH OF THE FOLLOWING AREAS OF THE CEREBELLUM ARE CLASSICALLY REGARDED AS THE VESTIBULOCEREBELLUM?:
A. Central lobule
B. Folium
C. Pyramis
D. Culmen
E. Flocculonodular lobe
Ref. 7 - p. 428

280. A LARGE NUCLEAR MASS JUST DORSAL TO THE MEDIAL GENICULATE BODY IS THE:
A. Mammillary body
B. Red nucleus
C. Pulvinar
D. Substantia nigra
E. Habenular nucleus
Ref. 7 - p. 443

281. LOCATED BETWEEN THE PULVINAR AND CAUDATE NUCLEUS IS A FIBER BUNDLE CALLED THE:
A. Induseum griseum
B. Stria terminalis
C. Fasciculus retroflexus
D. Stria medullaris
E. Crus of the fornix Ref. 7 - p. 445

282. THE HABENULAR NUCLEI ARE LOCATED:
A. Just rostral to interpeduncular nucleus
B. Adjacent to infundibular recess
C. Ventral to inferior colliculus
D. On the dorsomedial surfaces of thalami
E. In the mesencephalon Ref. 7 - p. 447

283. THE TENIA THALAMI IS LOCATED:
A. Between the thalamus and putamen
B. Between the anterior and ventral anterior nuclei of the thalamus
C. Between the dorsal thalamus and hypothalamus
D. Between the dorso-medial and ventral lateral nuclei of the thalamus
E. At the site of attachment of the roof of the 3rd ventricle to the thalamus Ref. 7 - p. 448

284. THE ZONA INCERTA IS LOCATED:
A. Between the alveus and the dentate gyrus
B. Between the external capsule and extreme capsule
C. On the dorsal surface of corpus callosum
D. Between medial and lateral nuclear groups of the thalamus
E. Between the subthalamic nucleus and the tegmental field
Ref. 7 - p. 448

285. THE MAMMILLOTHALAMIC TRACT ORIGINATES IN THE MAMMILLARY BODY AND TERMINATES IN THE __________ NUCLEI OF THE THALAMUS:
A. Anterior
B. Medial
C. Midline
D. Lateral
E. Ventral
Ref. 7 - p. 448

286. THE SUBTHALAMIC REGION CONTAINS ALL OF THE LISTED STRUCTURES, EXCEPT:
A. Subthalamic nucleus
B. Zona incerta
C. Stratum zonale
D. Lenticular fasciculus
E. Thalamic fasciculus
Ref. 7 - p. 452

287. THE SEPTUM PELLUCIDUM SEPARATES THE:
A. Thalamus from caudate nucleus
B. Thalamus from the globus pallidus
C. Putamen from cortex of insula
D. Left and right lateral ventricles
E. Left and right cerebral hemispheres Ref. 7 - p. 457

288. THE EPITHALAMUS DOES NOT INCLUDE:
A. The fornix
B. Pineal body
C. Habenular trigones
D. Epithelial roof of the III ventricle
E. Striae medullares Ref. 7 - p. 458

289. ALL OF THE LISTED NUCLEI FORM THE VENTRAL NUCLEAR GROUP OF THE THALAMUS, EXCEPT THE:
A. Ventral anterior nucleus
B. Ventral lateral nucleus
C. Ventral posterolateral nucleus
D. Ventral posteromedial nucleus
E. Anteroventral nucleus Ref. 7 - p. 460

290. ALL STATEMENTS ARE TRUE CONCERNING CONNECTIONS OF THE PULVINAR, EXCEPT:
A. Receives long ascending sensory fibers
B. Receives numerous connections from other thalamic nuclei
C. Projects to posterior parietal region
D. Projects to posterior parts of the temporal lobe
E. Projects to the area surrounding the striate cortex
Ref. 7 - p. 468

291. AFFERENT FIBERS TO THE VENTRAL ANTERIOR THALAMIC NUCLEUS ARISE FROM THE:
A. Globus pallidus
B. Red nucleus
C. Cerebellum
D. Occipital cortex
E. Spinal cord long ascending tracts Ref. 7 - p. 468

292. THE __________ NUCLEUS OF THE THALAMUS SERVES AS A RELAY NUCLEUS FOR CEREBELLAR IMPULSES REACHING THE PRECENTRAL CORTEX:
A. Ventral anterior
B. Ventral lateral
C. Ventral posterolateral
D. Ventral posteromedial
E. Dorsomedial
Ref. 7 - p. 469

293. ALL STATEMENTS CONCERNING CONNECTIONS OF THE VENTRAL POSTERIOR NUCLEUS ARE TRUE, EXCEPT:
A. The ventral posterolateral nucleus receives projections from the medial lemniscus
B. The ventral posterolateral nucleus receives projections from the spinothalamic tract
C. The ventral posterolateral nucleus contains the representation of the contralateral head, face and intraoral structures
D. Crossed and uncrossed secondary trigeminal fibers terminate in the ventral posteromedial nucleus
E. The ventral posterior nucleus has a precise topical projection to the cortex of the postcentral gyrus Ref. 7 - p. 470.

294. THE PRINCIPAL CORTICAL PROJECTION OF THE MEDIAL GENICULATE BODY IS TO THE:
A. Calcarine cortex
B. Superior temporal convolution
C. Precentral gyrus
D. Cingulate gyrus
E. Frontal lobe Ref. 7 - p. 472

295. THE LATERAL GENICULATE BODY HAS THE FOLLOWING CONNECTIONS,WITH THE EXCEPTION OF THE:
A. Optic tract
B. Calcarine cortex
C. Inferior colliculi
D. Pretectal area
E. Pulvinar, ventral and lateral thalamic nuclei
Ref. 7 - p. 472

296. THE THALAMIC RADIATIONS ARE USUALLY GROUPED INTO A NUMBER OF THALAMIC PEDUNCLES OR STALKS. ALL LISTED CONNECTIONS OF THE PEDUNCLES ARE CORRECT, EXCEPT:
A. Anterior or frontal peduncle connects the frontal lobe with the medial and anterior thalamic nuclei
B. The superior or centroparietal peduncle connects the rolandic area with the ventral thalamic nuclei
C. Posterior or occipital peduncle connects occipital and posterior parietal convolutions with caudal portions of the thalamus
D. Inferior or temporal peduncle connects the transverse temporal gyrus with the medial geniculate body
E. Medial thalamic peduncle represented by massa intermedia connects parietal lobe with medial nuclei of thalamus
Ref. 7 - p. 474

297. THE GENU OF THE INTERNAL CAPSULE CONTAINS THE__________ FIBERS:
A. Frontopontine
B. Corticobulbar
C. Corticospinal to lower extremity
D. Superior thalamic radiation
E. Corticorubral Ref. 7 - p. 476

298. THE POSTERIOR LIMB OF THE INTERNAL CAPSULE CONTAINS WHICH OF THE FOLLOWING?:
A. Superior thalamic radiations
B. Corticobulbar
C. Frontopontine fibers
D. Anterior
E. Corticospinal fibers Ref. 7 - p. 477

299. IDENTIFY THE STRUCTURE WHICH IS NOT PART OF THE VISUAL PATHWAY:
A. Rods and cones
B. Bipolar neurones
C. Ganglionic neurones
D. Optic nerve, chiasm and tract
E. Medial geniculate body Ref. 7 - p. 479

300. THE RETINAL AREAS HAVE THE FOLLOWING PRECISE RELATIONSHIPS WITH THE LATERAL GENICULATE BODY:
A. The upper retinal quadrants project to the medial half of the lateral geniculate body
B. Lower retinal quadrants project to the inferior part of the lateral geniculate body
C. Nasal retinal quadrants project to the medial half of the lateral geniculate body
D. Temporal retinal quadrants project to the lateral half of the lateral geniculate body
E. Macular fibers terminate in the 1, 3 and 6 laminae of the lateral geniculate body
Ref. 7 - p. 480

301. THE MEDIAL HALF OF THE LATERAL GENICULATE BODY PROJECTS TO THE__________OF THE CEREBRAL CORTEX:
A. Superior lip of the calcarine sulcus
B. Inferior lip of the calcarine sulcus
C. Caudal third of the calcarine cortex
D. Rostral portions of the calcarine cortex
E. Rostral portion of the lingual gyrus
Ref. 7 - p. 480

302. THE SPECIFIC SENSORY RELAY NUCLEI OF THE THALAMUS ARE LOCATED IN WHICH TIER OF THE LATERAL NUCLEAR GROUP?:
A. Ventral
B. Dorsal
C. Anterior
D. Posterior
E. None of the above
Ref. 7 - p. 482

303. THE THALAMUS IS A SUBCORTICAL CENTER FOR RECOGNITION OF:
A. Two point discrimination
B. Olfaction
C. Proprioception
D. Crude awareness of touch, temperature and pain
E. Sense of position
Ref. 7 - p. 483

304. THE ASSOCIATION NUCLEI OF THE THALAMUS RECEIVE NO DIRECT FIBERS FROM WHICH OF THE FOLLOWING?:
A. Hypothalamus
B. Epithalamus
C. Mammillary bodies
D. Habenular nuclei
E. Ascending systems
Ref. 7 - p. 485

305. IN THE HYPOTHALAMUS THE FORNIX SEPARATES:
A. The lateral preoptic area from the supraoptic nucleus
B. Posterior hypothalamic nucleus from the ventromedial hypothalamic nucleus
C. Lateral hypothalamic area from the lateral mammillary nucleus
D. Nuclei tuberis from the lateral hypothalamic nucleus
E. Medial and lateral hypothalamic areas
Ref. 7 - p. 488

306. THE SUPRAOPTIC REGION OF THE HYPOTHALAMUS CONTAINS THE:
A. Dorsomedial nucleus
B. Ventromedial nucleus
C. Mammillary body
D. Paraventricular nucleus
E. Posterior nucleus Ref. 7 - p. 489

307. NEUROSECRETORY CELLS ARE RECOGNIZED IN THE__________ NUCLEI OF THE HYPOTHALAMUS:
A. Dorsomedial and ventromedial
B. Tuberal
C. Medial and lateral mammillary
D. Lateral and posterior
E. Supraoptic and paraventricular Ref. 7 - p. 489

308. THE FIBERS FORMING THE MEDIAL FOREBRAIN BUNDLE ARISE FROM ALL THE AREAS LISTED BELOW, EXCEPT:
A. Cells in the basal olfactory regions
B. Cells in the periamygdaloid region
C. The cells in the septal nuclei
D. The cells in the paraventricular nucleus
Ref. 7 - p. 491

309. THE HIPPOCAMPO-HYPOTHALAMIC FIBERS THAT FORM THE FORNIX TERMINATE LARGELY IN THE:
A. Posterior hypothalamic nucleus
B. Medial mammillary nucleus
C. Lateral mammillary nucleus
D. Lateral hypothalamic nucleus
E. Supraoptic nucleus Ref. 7 - p. 491

310. THE MAJORITY OF FIBERS FORMING THE MAMMILLARY PEDUNCLE ARISE FROM CELLS OF THE:
A. Dorsal and ventral tegmental nuclei
B. Lateral mammillary nucleus
C. Medial mammillary nucleus
D. Paraventricular and posterior hypothalamic nuclei
E. Habenular nuclei Ref. 7 - p. 493

311. ALL STATEMENTS CONCERNING COMPOSITION OF THE FASCICULUS MAMMILLARIS PRINCEPS ARE TRUE, EXCEPT:
A. Divides into the mammillothalamic tract and the mammillotegmental tract
B. The mammillothalamic fibers originate from the medial and lateral mammillary nuclei
C. The mammillothalamic fibers terminate in the ipsilateral ventrolateral nucleus of the thalamus
D. The mammillotegmental fibers curve caudally into the midbrain tegmentum
E. Fibers of the mammillotegmental tract terminate in the dorsal and ventral tegmental nuclei Ref. 7 - p. 494

312. HYPOTHALAMIC REGIONS CONCERNED WITH THE CONTROL OF THE SYMPATHETIC RESPONSES ARE THE:
A. Lateral and posterior nuclei
B. Anterior nuclei
C. Dorsomedian and ventromedial nuclei
D. Paraventricular and supraoptic nuclei
E. Preoptic and tuberal nuclei Ref. 7 - p. 495

313. MAINTENANCE OF BODY WATER BALANCE IS RELATED TO THE __________NUCLEI OF THE HYPOTHALAMUS:
A. Supraoptic and paraventricular
B. Tuberal and mammillary
C. Dorsomedian and ventrolateral
D. Lateral and posterior
E. Anterior Ref. 7 - p. 495

314. THE FEEDING CENTER IS LOCATED IN THE__________HYPOTHALAMIC NUCLEUS:
A. Anterior
B. Lateral
C. Dorsomedial
D. Paraventricular
E. Tuberal
Ref. 7 - p. 497

315. THE MORE PROMINENT FIBER BUNDLES OF THE SUBTHALAMUS INCLUDE WHICH OF THE FOLLOWING?:
A. Ansa lenticularis
B. Fasciculus lenticularis
C. Thalamic fasciculus
D. Fornix
E. Stria medullaris
Ref. 7 - p. 497

316. THE__________HYPOTHALAMIC AREA IS SENSITIVE TO INCREASES IN TEMPERATURE:
A. Posterior
B. Anterior
C. Medial
D. Lateral
E. Tuberal
Ref. 7 - p. 496

317. ALL THE LISTED STRUCTURES ARE PART OF THE SUBTHALAMUS, EXCEPT THE:
A. Tegmental field of Forel
B. Ansa lenticularis
C. Fasciculus lenticularis
D. Subthalamic nucleus
E. Mammillary bodies Ref. 7 - p. 497

318. THE BASAL GANGLIA DO NOT INCLUDE THE:
A. Caudate nucleus
B. Putamen
C. Globus pallidus
D. Subthalamic nucleus
E. Amygdaloid complex
Ref. 7 - p. 498

319. THE AMYGDALOID NUCLEAR COMPLEX IS LOCATED IN THE:
A. Temporal lobe
B. Parietal lobe
C. Diencephalon
D. Cerebellum
E. Hypothalamus
Ref. 7 - p. 498

320. THE ANATOMICALLY WELL-DEFINED AFFERENT CONNECTIONS OF THE AMYGDALOID COMPLEX ORIGINATE IN THE:
A. Olfactory bulb
B. Cerebellar cortex
C. Anterior thalamus
D. Basal ganglia
E. Parietal lobe
Ref. 7 - p. 499

321. THE MOST PROMINENT EFFERENT PATHWAY FROM THE AMYGDALOID COMPLEX IS THE:
A. Fornix
B. Stria terminalis
C. Stria medullaris
D. Cingulum
E. Lenticular fasciculus
Ref. 7 - p. 499

322. THE CLAUSTRUM IS A PLATE OF GRAY MATTER LOCATED:
A. On the dorsal surface of the corpus callosum
B. On the surface of the dentate gyrus
C. In the calcarine sulcus
D. In the subthalamic area
E. Between external and extreme capsules
Ref. 7 - p. 501

323. THE CORPUS STRIATUM IS FORMED BY:
A. Amygdaloid nucleus and putamen
B. Thalamus and caudate nucleus
C. Lenticular nucleus and caudate nucleus
D. Putamen and globus pallidus
E. Subthalamic nucleus and globus pallidus
Ref. 7 - p. 501

324. THE CAUDATE NUCLEUS IS LOCATED:
A. Inferiorly and lateral to the internal capsule
B. Lateral to the thalamus
C. Medial to the globus pallidus
D. In the ventricular surface of the lateral ventricle
E. In the ventricular surface of the third ventricle
Ref. 7 - p. 501

325. STRIATAL AFFERENT FIBERS DO NOT INCLUDE:
A. Corticostriate fibers
B. Thalamostriate fibers
C. Nigrostriate fibers
D. Hypothalmostriate fibers
E. Striopallidal
Ref. 7 - p. 505

326. THE PALLIDO EFFERENT FIBERS DO NOT INCLUDE THE:
A. Lenticular fasciculus
B. Ansa lenticularis
C. Pallidotegmental fibers
D. Pallidosubthalamic fibers
E. Pallidospinal fibers
Ref. 7 - p. 506

327. PALLIDOFUGAL FIBERS WHICH TRAVERSE THE VENTRAL PART OF THE INTERNAL CAPSULE ARE THE:
A. Ansa lenticularis
B. Lenticular fasciculus
C. Thalamic fasciculus
D. Pallidotegmental fibers
E. Pallidosubthalamic fibers Ref. 7 - p. 507

328. THE EXTRAPYRAMIDAL SYSTEM SUBSERVES__________FUNCTIONS:
A. Visceral motor
B. Somatic motor
C. Special visceral motor
D. Special somatic sensory
E. Special visceral sensory Ref. 7 - p. 512

329. THE EXTRAPYRAMIDAL MOTOR SYSTEM INCLUDES WHICH OF THE FOLLOWING?:
A. Subthalamic nuclei
B. Habenular nuclei
C. Substantia nigra
D. Internal capsule
E. Red nucleus
Ref. 7 - p. 512

330. THE PRE-RUBRAL FIELD CONTAINS WHICH OF THE FOLLOWING?:
A. Zona incerta
B. Amygdala
C. Nucleus campi foreli
D. Corpus Luysi
E. Pallidofugal fibers Ref. 7 - p. 512

331. THE OLFACTORY LOBE MAKES ITS APPEARANCE DURING THE__________MONTH OF FETAL DEVELOPMENT:
A. 4th
B. 6th
C. 2nd
D. 9th
E. 5th
Ref. 7 - p. 518

332. RHINENCEPHALON WHICH RECEIVES FIBERS FROM THE OLFACTORY BULB DOES NOT INCLUDE THE:
A. Olfactory tubercle and striae
B. Anterior olfactory nucleus
C. Parts of the amygdaloid complex
D. Prepyriform cortex
E. Hippocampal formation Ref. 7 - p. 518

333. THE ARCHIPALLIUM, THE OLDEST CORTICAL DERIVATIVE, IS REPRESENTED BY THE FOLLOWING STRUCTURES, EXCEPT THE:
A. Hippocampal formation
B. Dentate gyrus
C. Olfactory bulb
D. Fasciolar gyrus
E. Indusium griseum
Ref. 7 - p. 518

334. THE CORTICAL PART OF THE SEPTAL AREA INCLUDES THE:
A. Olfactory bulb
B. Septum pellucidum
C. Subcallosal area and the paraterminal gyrus
D. Dentate gyrus
E. Parahippocampal gyrus Ref. 7 - p. 520

335. THE LATERAL OLFACTORY STRIA TERMINATE IN ALL THE LISTED STRUCTURES, EXCEPT THE:
A. Uncus
B. Parahippocampal gyrus
C. Amygdaloid nucleus
D. Prepyriform area
E. Stria terminalis
Ref. 7 - p. 522

336. WHICH OF THE FOLLOWING STATEMENTS CONCERNING THE OLFACTORY NERVE IS INCORRECT?:
A. Conducts special afferent impulses
B. The cell bodies of the sensory neuron are located in the olfactory bulb
C. The olfactory fila pass through the cribriform plate of the ethmoid bone
D. The olfactory fila represent the central processes of bipolar cells in the olfactory epithelium
E. The olfactory sensory cells have a coarse peripheral process from which short olfactory hairs arise projecting onto the surface of the olfactory epithelium Ref. 7 - p. 524

337. MITRAL CELLS ARE CHARACTERISTIC OF THE:
A. Cerebellar cortex
B. Primary visual cortex
C. Gray matter of the olfactory bulb
D. Primary somesthetic cortex
E. Primary motor cortex Ref. 7 - p. 524

338. ALL OF THE FOLLOWING STATEMENTS CONCERNING FIBER DISTRIBUTION OF THE ANTERIOR COMMISSURE ARE TRUE, EXCEPT:
A. Compact fiber bundle passing immediately in front of the anterior columns of the fornix
B. Laterally splits into a small anterior and larger posterior portion
C. The anterior portion connects the gray substance of the olfactory tract on one side with the olfactory bulb of the opposite side
D. The posterior portion mainly interconnects the middle temporal gyri
E. The posterior portion interconnects the habenular nuclei
Ref. 7 - p. 527

339. WHICH OF THE FOLLOWING STATEMENTS CONCERNING DISTRIBUTION OF THE DENTATE GYRUS IS INCORRECT?:
A. It is located between the collateral sulcus and the hippocampal fissure
B. It is continuous with the fasciolar gyrus
C. It spreads out into indusium griseum or supracallosal gyrus
D. It is continuous with the median and lateral longitudinal striae
E. Through structures listed above it becomes continuous with the paraterminal gyrus Ref. 7 - p. 530

340. THE CORTEX OF THE HIPPOCAMPAL FORMATION HAS __________ LAYERS:
A. 6
B. 5
C. 4
D. 3
E. 2 Ref. 7 - p. 531

341. ALL OF THE FOLLOWING STATEMENTS CONCERNING DISPOSITION OF FIBERS IN THE FORNIX ARE TRUE, EXCEPT THAT:
A. It is the main efferent fiber system of the hippocampal formation
B. They contain projection and commissural fibers
C. They originate from large pyramidal cells which form the alveus and fimbria
D. They reach the splenium of the corpus callosum as the crura of the fornix
E. All fibers decussate in the fornical commissure and continue as the body of the fornix Ref. 7 - p. 535

342. FIBERS OF THE FORNIX TERMINATE IN ALL THE LISTED AREAS, EXCEPT:
A. Postcommissural fibers in the mammillary body
B. Postcommissural fibers in the thalamus
C. Precommissural fibers in the septal area
D. Precommissural fibers in the lateral preoptic area and the hypothalamus
E. Precommissural fibers in the olfactory bulb and amygdaloid complex
Ref. 7 - p. 536

343. SPECIFICALLY, THE LIMBIC LOBE DOES NOT INCLUDE THE:
A. Subcallosal gyrus
B. Cingulate gyrus
C. Parahippocampal gyri
D. Hippocampal formation and dentate gyrus
E. Insular cortex Ref. 7 - p. 538

344. PROCEEDING FROM THE SURFACE OF THE CORTEX TOWARDS THE MEDULLARY SUBSTANCE, THE EXTERNAL PYRAMIDAL LAYER IS THE_________ LAYER IN THE NEOPALLIAL CORTEX:
A. First
B. Second
C. Third
D. Fourth
E. Fifth
Ref. 7 - p. 546

345. THE FOLLOWING CELLS ARE FOUND IN THE CEREBRAL NEOCORTEX, EXCEPT THE:
A. Purkinje cells
B. Pyramidal cells
C. Stellate or granule cells
D. Fusiform or spindle cells
E. Horizontal cells of Cajal and the cells of Martinotti
Ref. 7 - p. 543

346. THE EXTERNAL BAND OF BAILLARGER CONSIDERED TO BE THE TERMINAL RAMIFICATION OF THALAMOCORTICAL FIBERS IS LOCATED IN THE_________ LAYER OF THE NEOCORTEX:
A. I
B. II
C. III
D. IV
E. V Ref. 7 - p. 546

347. ACCORDING TO ECONOMO'S CLASSIFICATION, AN AGRANULAR TYPE OF CORTEX IS CHARACTERISTIC OF:
A. Precentral gyrus
B. Parietal cortex
C. Frontal pole
D. Calcarine cortex
E. Inferior temporal gyrus Ref. 7 - p. 553

348. THE PRIMARY SOMESTHETIC AREA IN THE CEREBRAL CORTEX CONSISTS OF THE:
A. Inferior frontal gyrus
B. Postcentral gyrus and its medial extension into paracentral lobule
C. Precentral gyrus
D. Superior temporal gyrus
E. Supramarginal gyrus Ref. 7 - p. 555

349. THE SECONDARY VISUAL AREA OF THE CEREBRAL CORTEX IS NUMBER__________ACCORDING TO THE BRODMANN CLASSIFICATION:
A. 3
B. 6
C. 8
D. 18
E. 22
Ref. 7 - p. 557

350. THE "SENSORY HOMUNCULUS" REPRESENT VARIOUS REGIONS OF THE BODY IN SPECIFIC PORTIONS OF THE POSTCENTRAL GYRUS. IDENTIFY THE BODY AREA OUT OF ORDER IN THE PATTERN OF REPRESENTATION:
A. The face area lies most ventral
B. Above face area is the leg area
C. Higher is the hand
D. Higher is the trunk
E. Last is the foot extending into paracentral lobule
Ref. 7 - p. 558

351. THE PREMOTOR AREA IS DESIGNATED AS AREA:
A. 3
B. 1
C. 2
D. 4
E. 6
Ref. 7 - p. 573

352. THE FRONTAL EYE FIELD RESPONSIBLE FOR VOLUNTARY SCANNING MOVEMENTS OF THE EYES IS REPRESENTED IN CORTICAL AREAS:
A. 3, 1, 2
B. 6
C. 4
D. 8
E. 19
Ref. 7 - p. 577

353. WHICH OF THE FOLLOWING ARE CHARACTERISTIC OF THE ELECTRICAL ACTIVITY OF SLOW SLEEP ?:
A. High voltage slow waves
B. Low voltage fast activity
C. High voltage fast activity
D. Low voltage slow waves
E. None of the above Ref. 7 - p. 584

354. PARADOXICAL SLEEP HAS WHICH OF THE FOLLOWING BEHAVIORAL CHARACTERISTICS?:
A. Spinal reflex activity is increased
B. Reduction in blood pressure
C. Bursts of rapid eye movements
D. Bradycardia
E. Increased muscle tone in neck muscles
Ref. 7 - p. 584

355. THE PREOPTIC AREA IS:
A. Divided into medial and lateral nuclei
B. Anterior to the lamina terminalis
C. Connected to the parolfactory area and the nucleus of the diagonal band
D. Posterior to the anterior hypothalamic area
E. Found in the tuber cinereum
Ref. 8 - p. 318

356. THE SUPRAOPTIC NUCLEUS:
A. Contains cells which send their axons into the anterior lobe of the hypophysis
B. Is composed of cells histologically similar to those of the paraventricular nucleus
C. Has a neurosecretory function
D. Lies above the rostral ends of the optic tract
E. Is also called the nucleus intercalatus
Ref. 8 - p. 319

357. THE SUPRAOPTIC REGION CONTAINS TWO OF THE MOST STRIKING AND SHARPLY DEFINED HYPOTHALAMIC NUCLEI WHICH INCLUDES WHICH OF THE FOLLOWING?:
A. Paraventricular
B. Lateral mammillary
C. Preoptic
D. Dorsomedial
E. Supraoptic
Ref. 7 - p. 489

358. THE MEDIAL FOREBRAIN BUNDLE:
A. Is large and conspicuous in man
B. Arises from the olfactory regions and septal nuclei
C. Passes through the lateral parts of the hypothalamus
E. Connects the thalamus with the subthalamus
E. Continues caudally into the midbrain tegmentum
Ref. 7 - p. 491

359. FIBERS OF THE FORNIX PROJECT MAINLY TO WHICH OF THE FOLLOWING NUCLEI?:
A. Dorsomedial nucleus
B. Anterior hypothalamic
C. Medial mammillary nucleus
D. Preoptic nucleus
E. Posterior hypothalamic nucleus
Ref. 7 - p. 491

360. THE AMYGDALOHYPOTHALAMIC FIBERS FOLLOW WHICH OF THE FOLLOWING PATHWAYS TO THE HYPOTHALAMUS?:
A. Fornix
B. Stria medullaris
C. A course ventral to the lentiform nucleus
D. Medial forebrain bundle
E. Stria terminalis
Ref. 7 - p. 492

361. THE MAMMILLOTHALAMIC TRACT:
A. Connects the mammillary bodies with the pulvinar
B. Is also called the Vicq d'Azyr bundle
C. Projects to the ventral tegmental nucleus
D. Passes from the mammillary bodies to the anterior thalamic nucleus
E. May be demonstrated by gross dissection
Ref. 9 - p. 320

362. THE LATERAL CEREBRAL FISSURE:
A. Divides into three branches lateralward
B. Separates the frontal and parietal lobes, which lie dorsal to it, from the temporal lobe
C. May be called the fissure of Rolando
D. Extends laterally as the parieto-occipital fissure
E. Separates the right and left cerebral hemispheres
Ref. 12 - p. 56

363. THE INSULA:
A. Overlies the corpus striatum
B. May be called the Island of Reil
C. Is hidden from view at the bottom of the lateral fissure
D. Is not well-developed in adults
E. Is without cortex
Ref. 12 - p. 59

364. THE NAME GYRUS FORNICATUS INCLUDES WHICH OF THE FOLLOWING?:
A. Uncus
B. Gyrus rectus
C. Gyrus cinguli
D. Precuneus
E. Hippocampal gyrus
Ref. 12 - p. 62

365. AT THE BOTTOM OF THE LONGITUDINAL FISSURE OF THE CEREBRUM IS A BROAD WHITE BAND OF COMMISSURAL FIBERS KNOWN AS THE:
A. Anterior commissure
B. Posterior commissure
C. Centrum semiovale
D. Fusiform gyrus
E. Corpus callosum
Ref. 12 - p. 63

366. THE CORPUS CALLOSUM IS SEEN TO BE ARCHED DORSALLY AND TO BE RELATED ON ITS VENTRAL SURFACE TO WHICH OF THE FOLLOWING?:
A. Septum pellucidum
B. Gyrus rectus
C. Collateral fissure
D. Calcar avis
E. Fornix
Ref. 12 - p. 63

367. THE RUDIMENTARY PORTION OF THE HIPPOCAMPUS IS KNOWN AS WHICH OF THE FOLLOWING?:
A. Tapetum
B. Forceps major
C. Supracallosal gyrus
D. Indusium griseum
E. Forceps minor
Ref. 12 - p. 65

368. THE LENTICULAR NUCLEUS INCLUDES WHICH OF THE FOLLOWING?:
A. Caudate nucleus
B. Claustrum
C. Putamen
D. Globus pallidus
E. Amygdaloid
Ref. 9 - p. 356

369. THE TAIL OF THE CAUDATE NUCLEUS EXTENDS FORWARD IN THE INFERIOR HORN TO FUSE WITH WHICH OF THE FOLLOWING?:
A. Claustrum
B. Globus pallidus
C. Amygdala
D. Thalamus
E. Hypothalamus
Ref. 9 - p. 361

370. THE LENTICULAR FASCICULUS:
A. Is often called the H_2 bundle of Forel
B. May be designated as the dorsal division of the ansa lenticularis
C. Arises from the globus pallidus
D. Arises from the caudate nucleus
E. Swings medialward across the anterior limb of the internal capsule to enter the cerebellum
Ref. 9 - p. 374

371. THE ANSA LENTICULARIS:
A. Receives fibers from various cortical areas
B. Projects primarily to the position occupied by the lenticular fasciculus
C. Arises primarily from the thalamus
D. Receives contributions from the substantia innominata
E. Arises from the putamen and both portions of the globus pallidus
Ref. 9 - p. 376

372. THE CLAUSTRUM:
A. Lies deep to the cortex of the Island of Reil
B. Is separated from the cortex of the insula by the external capsule
C. Is usually divisible into relatively distinct dorsal and ventral portions
D. Lies between the internal and external capsules
E. Is connected with the superior and middle temporal convolutions
Ref. 9 - p. 388

373. THE AMYGDALA IS:
A. Generally separated into two major divisions
B. Fused with the head of the caudate nucleus
C. Partly overlaid by the periamygdaloid cortex of the hippocampal gyrus
D. Found between the external and extreme capsules
E. Connected with the thalamus by way of the ansa lenticularis
Ref. 9 - p. 388

374. THE CORTICOMEDIAL PORTION OF THE AMYGDALOID COMPLEX:
A. Receives fibers from the lateral olfactory tract
B. Is larger than the basolateral subdivision of the human amygdala
C. Sends fibers to the parolfactory area by way of the stria medullaris
D. Has short internuclear connections with the basolateral nuclei
E. Is interconnected with the overlying cortex of the hippocampal gyrus
Ref. 9 - p. 390

375. WHICH OF THE FOLLOWING FIBER TRACTS PASS THROUGH THE ANTERIOR LIMB OF THE INTERNAL CAPSULE?:
A. Corticobulbar
B. Corticospinal
C. Frontopontine fibers
D. Auditory radiations
E. Anterior thalamic radiations
Ref. 9 - p. 396

376. WHICH OF THE FOLLOWING FIBER TRACTS PASS THROUGH THE SUBLENTICULAR PORTION OF THE POSTERIOR LIMB OF THE INTERNAL CAPSULE?:
A. Frontopontine fibers
B. Corticobulbar
C. Auditory radiations
D. Visual radiations
E. Cortico nigral
Ref. 9 - p. 397

377. ASSOCIATION FIBERS OF THE TELENCEPHALON INCLUDE WHICH OF THE FOLLOWING?:
A. Hippocampal commissure
B. Anterior commissure
C. Corpus callosum
D. Uncinate fasciculus
E. Cingulum
Ref. 9 - p. 404

378. THE AVERAGE THICKNESS OF THE CEREBRAL CORTEX IS APPROXIMATELY:
A. 1 mm
B. 2.5 mm
C. 5 mm
D. 3.5 mm
E. 4.5 mm
Ref. 9 - p. 410

379. CORTEX WHICH, ONTOGENETICALLY, SHOWS A SIX-LAYERED PATTERN OF LAMINATION HAS BEEN TERMED:
A. Homogenetic cortex
B. Heterogenetic cortex
C. Allocortex
D. Paleopallium
E. Isocortex
Ref. 9 - p. 410

380. EXCEPT FOR THE OLFACTORY CORTEX, THE PRIMARY SENSORY CORTICES RECEIVE THEIR MAIN INPUT FROM WHICH OF THE FOLLOWING?:
A. Hypothalamus
B. Thalamic relay nuclei
C. Basal ganglia
D. Red nucleus
E. Claustrum
Ref. 6 - p. 240

381. THE MOLECULAR LAYER OF CEREBRAL CORTEX SHOWS THE FOLLOWING CHARACTERISTICS:
A. Tangential myelinated fibers
B. Horizontal cells of Cajal
C. Large pyramidal cells
D. Irregular fusiform cells
E. Is the most superficial
Ref. 12 - p. 351

382. THE KONIOCORTEX INCLUDES WHICH OF THE FOLLOWING?:
A. Precentral gyrus
B. Brodmann area 4
C. Visual cortex
D. Auditory cortex
E. Postcentral gyrus
Ref. 12 - p. 353

383. USING CYTOARCHITECTURE AS A BASIS, BRODMANN HAS SUBDIVIDED THE HUMAN CORTEX INTO__________AREAS:
A. 52
B. 21
C. 105
D. 33
E. 78
Ref. 8 - p. 348

384. THE MOST POSTERIOR PART OF THE PYRIFORM LOBE IS THE ENTORHINAL AREA DESIGNATED AS AREA_________BY BRODMANN:
A. 41
B. 17
C. 4
D. 24
E. 28
Ref. 8 - p. 534

385. THE_________NUCLEI CONTRIBUTE AXONS TO THE STRIA MEDULLARIS:
A. Nucleus of the diagonal band of Broca
B. Vestibular
C. Septal
D. Red
E. Preoptic
Ref. 8 - p. 538

386. THE PREMOTOR CORTEX INCLUDES AREAS:
A. 6.
B. 17.
C. 8.
D. 44.
E. 3.
Ref. 6 - p. 245

387. THE TRANSVERSE GYRI OF HESCHL COMPRISE THE PRIMARY _________CORTEX:
A. Motor
B. Auditory
C. Visual
D. Premotor
E. Olfactory
Ref. 6 - p. 243

388. THE SOMESTHETIC ASSOCIATION CORTEX OF THE PARIETAL LOBE INCLUDES WHICH OF THE FOLLOWING AREAS?:
A. 7
B. 5
C. 17
D. 41
E. 18
Ref. 6 - p. 241

389. THE MOST PROMINENT OF THE PROCESSING STATIONS OF THE LIMBIC SYSTEM INCLUDES WHICH OF THE FOLLOWING?:
A. Caudate nucleus
B. Globus pallidus
C. Putamen
D. Hippocampal formation
E. Amygdala
Ref. 6 - p. 224

390. THE SUBSTANTIA NIGRA RECEIVES ITS MAIN INPUT FROM WHICH OF THE FOLLOWING AREAS?:
A. Cerebral cortex
B. Thalamus
C. Subthalamic nuclei
D. Globus pallidus
E. Red nucleus
Ref. 6 - p. 217

ANSWER THE FOLLOWING QUESTIONS (T)RUE OR (F)ALSE:

391. The hypothalamus is thought of as receiving its major input from the specific lemniscal system. Ref. 6 - p. 167

392. There are approximately three times as many cerebellar afferent fibers as cerebellar efferent fibers. Ref. 6 - p. 148

393. The middle cerebellar peduncle conveys information primarily from the pons. Ref. 6 - p. 148

394. The general somatic efferent cranial nerves have their nuclei of origin adjacent to the midline. Ref. 6 - p. 141

395. The pain and temperature fibers from the head are conveyed chiefly via the seventh cranial nerve. Ref. 6 - p. 134

396. The glossopharyngeal nerve conveys taste sensations from the posterior third of the tongue. Ref. 6 - p. 118

397. There is little if any overlapping between any two adjacent dermatomes. Ref. 6 - p. 83

398. The fifth cranial nerve innervates the tensor tympani muscle. Ref. 6 - p. 124

399. The juxtarestiform body consists of the fibers associated with the vestibular system, archicerebellum, and nuclei fastigii. Ref. 6 - p. 148

400. The superior cerebellar peduncle consists primarily of the efferent fibers from the dentate, emboliform, and globose nuclei. Ref. 6 - p. 149

SELECT THE MOST APPROPRIATE ANSWER(S):

401. THE SO-CALLED DISC OF MERKEL:
A. Terminates primarily in hairy skin
B. Is a somewhat specialized type of free nerve ending
C. Is covered by a capsule of connective tissue rich in fibrils, arranged in concentric lamellae
D. Encloses a protoplasmic bulb
E. Is frequently found in ligaments Ref. 1 - p. 33

402. THE PACINIAN CORPUSCLE:
A. May be seen only with the aid of a microscope
B. Is seldom found in the periosteum
C. Essentially records vibration
D. Shows no regressive changes with advancing age
E. May be classified as an unencapsulated nerve ending Ref. 1 - p. 38

403. MEISSNER'S CORPUSCLES:
A. Are found in the muscle spindles
B. Are expecially abundant where sensitiveness is highly developed
C. Run parallel to the hair shaft and terminate in the outer root sheath
D. Are found in the epithelial layers
E. Are elongated, elliptical formations with rounded ends, located in the cutaneous papillae Ref. 2 - p. 332

404. NERVE ENDINGS IN CARDIAC MUSCLE:
A. Belong to the myelinated fibers
B. Form motor end-plates
C. Have a more complex structure than those of skeletal muscles
D. End within the muscle fibers
E. Pass between the muscle trabeculae and appear to form no specialized contacts Ref. 2 - p. 328

405. THE ANNULOSPIRAL ENDINGS:
A. Function as stretch receptors
B. Are found in smooth muscle
C. Probably give rise to pain sensation
D. Are located at the junction of muscle fibers and their tendons
E. May also be called flower-spray endings
Ref. 2 - p. 330

406. WHICH OF THE FOLLOWING MAY BE COMMONLY CLASSIFIED AS PRESSURE RECEPTORS?:
A. Meissner's corpuscles
B. Merkel's discs
C. Free nerve endings
D. Pacinian corpuscles
E. Corpuscle of Ruffini
Ref. 3 - p. 965

407. WHICH OF THE FOLLOWING MAY COMMONLY BE CLASSIFIED AS PAIN RECEPTORS?:
A. Vater-pacinian corpuscles
B. Meissner's corpuscles
C. Flower-spray endings
D. Free nerve endings
E. Krause end-bulb
Ref. 3 - p. 966

408. THE PROPRIOCEPTIVE RECEPTORS OF STRIATED MUSCLES:
A. Include Herbst corpuscles
B. Include specially modified and encapsulated muscle fibers
C. May be found in abundance in most muscles but only rarely in the muscles of the extremity
D. Include the end-bulbs of Krause
E. Do not exist in the muscles of mastication
Ref. 4 - p. 240

409. THE NUCLEUS OF A NEURON USUALLY HAS THE FOLLOWING CHARACTERISTICS:
A. Small
B. Spherical or slightly ovoid
C. Usually centrally placed
D. Contains several nucleoli
E. Uniform dispersion of the chromatin
Ref. 2 - p. 308

410. THE NEUROPLASM OF THE NEURON:
A. May also be called perikaryon
B. Contains the sex chromatin
C. Is crowded with filamentous, membranous and granular organelles
D. Does not extend into the cell processes
E. Is called axoplasm in the axon
Ref. 2 - pp. 308-309

411. WHICH OF THE FOLLOWING ORGANELLES ARE MOST CHARACTERISTICALLY INVOLVED IN CHROMATOLYSIS?:
A. Neurofibrils
B. Chromophilic substance
C. Golgi apparatus
D. Nissl bodies
E. Mitochondria
Ref. 2 - p. 311

412. NEURONAL MITOCHONDRIA SHOW THE FOLLOWING CHARACTERISTICS:
A. Generally smaller than those of non-nervous tissues
B. Seldom found in axon endings
C. Cristae are consistently transverse
D. Dense granules are always present in the inner mitochondrial chamber
E. May be demonstrated in fresh nerve cells by supravital staining
Ref. 2 - p. 312

413. GOLGI TYPE I NEURONS SHOW THE FOLLOWING CHARACTERISTICS:
A. Have short axons
B. Have long axons
C. Are especially numerous in the cerebral cortex
D. Join in the formation of craniospinal nerves
E. Are numerous in the retina
Ref. 2 - p. 317

414. MYELIN IS ELABORATED BY WHICH OF THE FOLLOWING CELLS?:
A. Satellite cells
B. Fibrous astrocytes
C. Microglia
D. Oligodendrocytes
E. Schwann cells
Ref. 2 - pp. 321, 336

415. FIBROUS ASTROCYTES SHOW WHICH OF THE FOLLOWING CHARACTERISTICS?:
A. Found chiefly in the gray substance of the brain
B. Found chiefly in the white substance of the brain
C. Forms myelin in the CNS
D. Often attached to the blood vessels by means of their processes
E. Long, thin, smooth and infrequently branching processes
Ref. 2 - p. 336

416. THE OLIGODENDROCYTES SHOW WHICH OF THE FOLLOWING CHARACTERISTICS?:
A. Are larger than the astrocytes
B. Have many thick processes
C. Form myelin in the CNS
D. Are regarded as the homologue of the neurilemmal cells of Schwann
E. Have been shown to exhibit rhythmic pulsatile movements in tissue cultures
Ref. 2 - p. 336

417. THE MICROGLIA SHOW WHICH OF THE FOLLOWING CHARACTERISTICS?:
A. Cell bodies appear smooth
B. Are scattered everywhere throughout the brain and spinal cord
C. Are mesodermal in origin
D. Large nuclei
E. Numerous processes
Ref. 2 - p. 337

418. THE CHIEF SOURCE OF TUMORS OF THE CENTRAL NERVOUS SYSTEM IS:
A. Neurons
B. Neuroglia
C. Satellite cells
D. Astrocytes
E. Purkinje's cells
Ref. 2 - p. 338

419. WHICH OF THE FOLLOWING CELLS STAIN REASONABLY SPECIFICALLY BY THE DEL RIO-HORTEGA METHOD?:
A. Fibrous astrocytes
B. Protoplasmic astrocytes
C. Oligodendrocytes
D. Microglia
E. Brain macrophages
Ref. 2 - p. 507

420. THE GOLD CHLORIDE SUBLIMATE TECHNIC OF CAJAL IS A REASONABLY SPECIFIC METALLIC STAIN FOR WHICH OF THE FOLLOWING CELLS?:
A. Fibrous astrocytes
B. Microglia
C. Protoplasmic astrocytes
D. Schwann cells
E. Oligodendrocytes
Ref. 3 - p. 503

421. SYNAPTIC VESICLES ARE USUALLY LOCATED IN:
A. The dendrites
B. The nucleus of the neuron
C. The same area as neurofilaments
D. Rounded terminal boutons
E. Mitochondria
Ref. 2 - p. 339

422. THE PRE- AND POSTSYNAPTIC SURFACE MEMBRANES ARE SEPARATED BY A NARROW EXTRACELLULAR CLEFT ABOUT ________ WIDE:
A. 1800Å
B. 850Å
C. 740Å
D. 1200Å
E. 200Å
Ref. 2 - p. 339

423. THE DENSE CORE VESICLES PROBABLY CONTAIN:
A. Acetylcholine
B. 5-Hydroxytryptamine
C. Noradrenaline
D. GABA
E. Glutamate
Ref. 3 - p. 500

424. SWOLLEN TERMINATIONS OF AXONS:
A. Contain no mitochondria
B. Are called boutons
C. Contain many neurofilaments
D. Are called end-bulbs
E. Contain many nissl bodies
Ref. 3 - p. 500

425. MOTOR END-PLATES MAY BE DEMONSTRATED:
A. By gold and silver impregnation
B. In smooth muscle
C. In striated muscle
D. By routine H & E Stain
E. In cardiac muscle
Ref. 3 - p. 569

426. THE RHOMBENCEPHALON IS SUBDIVIDED INTO THE ________ AND THE ________:
A. Telencephalon
B. Diencephalon
C. Metencephalon
D. Myelencephalon
E. Prosencephalon
Ref. 5 - p. 316

427. THE MYELENCEPHALON DEVELOPS INTO THE:
A. Pons
B. Cerebellum
C. Diencephalon
D. Mesencephalon
E. Medulla
Ref. 5 - p. 316

428. IN THE HUMAN EMBRYO THE NEURAL PLATE FIRST APPEARS IN THE:
A. 10th somite stage
B. 3rd somite stage
C. Late pre-somite stage
D. 15th somite stage
E. Early pre-somite stage
Ref. 5 - p. 316

429. SPONGIOBLASTS SEPARATE FROM THE LIMITING MEMBRANES TO GIVE ORIGIN TO:
A. Astrocytoblasts
B. Microglia
C. Ependymal cells
D. Neuroblasts
E. Astrocytes
Ref. 5 - p. 318

430. THE NEURAL CREST ARISES FROM:
A. Ependymal cells
B. Medulloblasts
C. Microglia
D. Specialized ectoderm
E. Spongioblasts
Ref. 5 - p. 320

431. WHICH OF THE FOLLOWING CELLS ARE POSSIBLY DEVELOPED FROM NEURAL CREST CELLS?:
A. Dorsal root ganglion cells
B. Astrocytes
C. Oligodendrocytes
D. Neurolemmal sheath cells
E. Sympathetic ganglion cells
Ref. 5 - p. 322

432. IN THE HUMAN CENTRAL NERVOUS SYSTEM MYELINATION COMMENCES IN THE:
A. First month of fetal life
B. 100 mm C.R. length stage
C. Fourth month of fetal life
D. 50 mm C.R. length stage
E. Eighth month of fetal life
Ref. 5 - p. 323

433. IN THE HUMAN CENTRAL NERVOUS SYSTEM MYELINATION IS NOT COMPLETED UNTIL THE:
A. Fifth year
B. Twelfth year
C. Ninth month of fetal life
D. Second or third year
E. Twenty-first year
Ref. 5 - p. 323

434. THE__________PART OF THE SPINAL CORD IS THE FIRST PORTION TO DEVELOP MYELIN:
A. Lumbar
B. Thoracic
C. Sacral
D. Cervical
E. Caudal
Ref. 5 - p. 323

435. THE POSTERIOR COLUMNS OF WHITE MATTER BEGIN TO BE MYELINATED AT THE:
A. Second month of fetal life
B. Fourth month of fetal life
C. Second year
D. Sixth month of fetal life
E. First year Ref. 5 - p. 323

436. THE SPINO-CEREBELLAR AND SPINO-THALAMIC TRACTS BEGIN TO BE MYELINATED AT THE:
A. Seventh month of fetal life
B. Second month of fetal life
C. First year
D. Fourth year
E. Second year Ref. 5 - p. 323

437. THE DESCENDING MOTOR TRACTS (PYRAMIDAL AND RUBROSPINAL) BEGIN TO ACQUIRE THEIR MYELIN SHEATHS DURING THE:
A. Ninth fetal month
B. Second year
C. Fourth fetal month
D. First year
E. Third fetal month Ref. 5 - p. 323

ANSWER THE FOLLOWING QUESTIONS (T)RUE OR (F)ALSE:

438. Degenerating myelin sheaths can be demonstrated with the so-called Marchi method. Ref. 1 - p. 14

439. The degenerating myelin sheaths appear as yellow dots or somewhat longer cylindrical particles when using the Marchi method. Ref. 1 - p. 15

440. The normal myelinated fibers are stained black with the Marchi stain. Ref. 1 - p. 15

441. In large myelinated fibers the impulses are propagated with a speed of some 75 to 100 m per second. Ref. 1 - p. 42

442. In the finest unmyelinated fibers the velocity is only 1.5 to 0.3 meters per second. Ref. 1 - p. 42

443. The fibers in the dorsal roots enter the spinal cord in the dorsolateral sulcus. Ref. 1 - p. 42

444. The fibers in the dorsal roots which enter the spinal cord laterally are large, thick and usually myelinated. Ref. 1 - p. 43

445. The fibers in the dorsal roots which enter the spinal cord medially are thin and mainly unmyelinated. Ref. 1 - p. 44

446. The nervous system is one of the first organ systems to function during embryonic life. Ref. 6 - p. 65

447. Up to about the eighth month, the spinal cord extends throughout the entire length of the developing vertebral column.
Ref. 6 - p. 68

448. At birth the caudal end of the spinal cord is located at the level of the third lumbar vertebra. Ref. 6 - p. 68

449. The adult spinal cord is located at the level approximately between the first and second lumbar vertebrae. Ref. 6 - p. 68

450. In the spinal cord, the sensory nuclei of the peripheral nerves become differentiated in the gray matter of the basal plate.
Ref. 6 - p. 68

SELECT THE MOST APPROPRIATE ANSWER(S):

451. THE PERIPHERAL NERVOUS SYSTEM DEVELOPS FROM THE FOLLOWING PRIMORDIAL SOURCES:
A. Alar plate neuroblasts
B. Endoderm
C. Undifferentiated mesoderm
D. Neuroblasts of the neural crest
E. Spongioblasts
Ref. 6 - p. 69

452. THE LARGE BRAIN IN THE NEWBORN INFANT EXCEEDS__________ PERCENT OF THE ENTIRE BODY WEIGHT:
A. 10
B. 20
C. 30
D. 25
E. 18
Ref. 6 - p. 70

453. IN THE ADULT THE BRAIN CONSTITUTES APPROXIMATELY __________PERCENT OF THE TOTAL BODY WEIGHT:
A. 10
B. 20
C. 8
D. 5
E. 2
Ref. 6 - p. 72

454. THE LENGTH OF THE NORMAL MALE ADULT SPINAL CORD FROM ITS UPPER LIMIT TO THE TIP OF THE CONUS MEDULLARIS IS ABOUT:
A. 24 cm
B. 38 cm
C. 18 cm
D. 80 cm
E. 45 cm
Ref. 7 - p. 27

455. THE LENGTH OF THE NORMAL MALE VERTEBRAL COLUMN IS ABOUT:
A. 30 cm
B. 80 cm
C. 100 cm
D. 70 cm
E. 50 cm
Ref. 7 - p. 27

456. THE FILUM TERMINALE:
A. Does not penetrate the dura
B. Is composed mainly of pial connective tissue
C. Is composed of nervous tissue
D. Terminates at the level of the second sacral vertebra
E. Is also called the conus medullaris
Ref. 7 - p. 27

457. THE SUBSTANTIA GLIOSA IS LOCATED IN THE:
A. Anterior columns
B. Posterior columns
C. Reticular formation
D. Gray commissure
E. Lateral funiculus
Ref. 7 - p. 29

458. THE SIXTH CERVICAL SPINOUS PROCESS OVERLIES THE:
A. Eighth cervical spinal cord segment
B. Sixth cervical spinal cord segment
C. Fourth cervical spinal cord segment
D. Second thoracic spinal cord segment
E. Fifth thoracic spinal cord segment Ref. 8 - p. 79

459. THE CENTRAL CANAL OF THE ADULT SPINAL CORD:
A. Is lined by ependyma
B. Usually contains fluid
C. Does not continue into the conus medullaris
D. Continues through the brain stem
E. Disappears after age 55 Ref. 8 - p. 79

460. THE DURA MATER SURROUNDING THE SPINAL CORD EXTENDS TO A LEVEL OPPOSITE THE:
A. Fourth lumbar vertebra
B. Second sacral vertebra
C. Twelfth thoracic vertebra
D. Second lumbar vertebra
E. Fifth sacral vertebra Ref. 8 - p. 80

461. THE SPINAL DURA IS USUALLY ATTACHED AT THE FOLLOWING AREAS:
A. Foramen magnum
B. Anterior longtiudinal ligament
C. Periosteum of the posterior surfaces of the second and third cervical vertebrae
D. Fourth sacral vertebra
E. Posterior longitudinal ligament Ref. 8 - p. 80

462. THE DENTICULATE LIGAMENT:
A. Extends laterally as a single-layered fold
B. Is arranged as a series of about 21 dentate processes
C. Attaches to the inner surface of the dura
D. Is formed from the arachnoid
E. Is formed from pia Ref. 8 - p. 81

463. THE FIRST PAIR OF SPINAL NERVES:
A. Exits from the vertebral column between the atlas and the axis
B. Carries no sympathetic fibers
C. Passes through the foramen magnum
D. Exits from the vertebral column between the atlas and the skull
E. Has no dorsal root ganglia Ref. 9 - p. 58

464. THE LUMBAR SEGMENTS OF THE ADULT CORD ARE AT APPROXIMATELY THE LEVELS OF THE SPINOUS PROCESSES OF:
A. T_{11} and T_{12}
B. L_2 and L_5
C. S_2 and S_5
D. T_5 and T_8
E. L_4 and L_5
Ref. 9 - p. 59

465. AS THE LIMB BUDS GROW OUT, THEY CARRY WITH THEM THE SEGMENTAL INNERVATION OF THE DERMATOMES WHICH INCLUDE:
A. C_1 to C_4
B. T_5 to L_1
C. L_2 to S_3
D. S_4 to S_5
E. C_4 to T_2
Ref. 9 - p. 59

466. THE EPINEURIUM:
A. Invests an entire nerve
B. Invests bundles within a nerve
C. Is the innermost of three traditional fibrous nerve sheaths
D. Consists of strands of coarse connective tissue which run chiefly lengthwise
E. Provides a tough protective coat for the nerve
Ref. 10 - p. 46

467. THE PERINEURIUM:
A. Is arranged chiefly in circular layers
B. Is continuous with the pia mater
C. Is located outside the epineurium
D. Has both an inner and outer layer of dense fibrous tissue
E. Offers a firm hold for sutures in nerve repairs
Ref. 10 - p. 47

ANSWER THE FOLLOWING QUESTIONS (T)RUE OR (F)ALSE:

468. Crushing injuries or interruption of an axon produces detectable changes in the cell body known as chromatolysis.
Ref. 7 - p. 139

469. Following an injury to an axon, the proximal portion of the fiber which is attached to the cell body shows some degree of retrograde degeneration.
Ref. 7 - p. 139

470. The distal portion of the injured axon disintegrates without any loss of the myelin sheath. Ref. 7 - p. 139

471. Schwann cells are almost exclusively responsible for the removal of axon remnants and autodigestion of disintegrated myelin.
Ref. 7 - p. 141

472. Numerous leucocytes appear to participate in the phagocytosis of neuronal debris. Ref. 7 - p. 141

473. Chromatolysis in the cell body reaches its maximum 12 to 14 days following injury to the axon. Ref. 7 - p. 144

474. Recovery in an injured nerve cell begins about the third week.
Ref. 7 - p. 144

475. Full recovery of an injured axon, depending on the mass of axon to be reconstituted, requires about 2 to 8 weeks.
Ref. 7 - p. 144

476. The leptomeninges include both the dura mater and arachnoid.
Ref. 7 - p. 12

477. The subdural space has no direct communication with the subarachnoid space.
Ref. 7 - p. 12

478. The diaphragma sellae forms the fibrous roof of the pituitary fossa.
Ref. 7 - p. 13

479. The dura mater receives its major blood supply through the foramen ovale.
Ref. 7 - p. 13

SELECT THE MOST APPROPRIATE ANSWER(S)

480. THE FORAMEN OF MAGENDIE:
A. Is located in the caudal part of the fourth ventricular roof
B. Is a median aperture
C. Is located in the lateral aspect of the fourth ventricle
D. Connects the lateral ventricles with the third ventricle
E. Is absent whenever the foramina of Luschka are present
Ref. 7 - p. 18

481. ARACHNOID GRANULATIONS ARE:
A. Simple prolongations of pia-arachnoid tissue which protrude into a venous sinus
B. Not visible with the naked eye
C. Most numerous along the interhemispheric fissure
D. Also called pacchionian bodies
E. Not observed in the spinal arachnoid Ref. 7 - p. 19

482. CEREBROSPINAL FLUID NORMALLY:
A. Contains large amounts of protein and glucose
B. Contains small amounts of potassium and sodium chloride
C. Appears pale yellow and highly cellular
D. Provides a fluid pathway for neural metabolites to be returned to the venous system
E. Has a specific gravity of 1.004 to 1.007
Ref. 7 - p. 20

483. IN MAN THE LUMBAR CEREBROSPINAL FLUID PRESSURE IN THE RECUMBENT POSITION IS NORMALLY:
A. 80-100 mm H_2O
B. 200-300 mm H_2O
C. 100-150 mm H_2O
D. 50-75 mm H_2O
E. 150-200 mm H_2O
Ref. 7 - p. 21

484. CIRCULATION OF CEREBROSPINAL FLUID IN THE VENTRICLES IS VULNERABLE TO BLOCKING AT WHICH OF THE FOLLOWING AREAS?:
A. Central canal
B. Interventricular foramen
C. Cerebral aqueduct
D. Foramina of Luschka
E. Virchow-Robin space
Ref. 10 - p. 428

485. THE CIRCULATION OF THE BRAIN AND SPINAL CORD DIFFERS FROM THAT OF OTHER ORGANS IN WHICH OF THE FOLLOWING ASPECTS?:
A. Veins and sinuses have valves
B. Venous return traces back the course of corresponding arteries
C. Cerebral arteries in general have very thin walls
D. Cerebral veins have thicker walls than do the cerebral arteries
E. Cerebral arteries have little elastic tissue and scanty smooth muscle
Ref. 10 - p. 433

486. THE VERTEBRAL ARTERIES:
A. Enter the skull via the foramen magnum
B. Unite at the caudal border of the pons to form the basilar artery
C. Enter the cavernous sinus
D. Give rise to the posterior inferior cerebellar arteries
E. Usually give rise to the superior cerebellar arteries
Ref. 10 - p. 434

487. THE INTERNAL CAROTID ARTERIES GIVE RISE TO WHICH OF THE FOLLOWING ARTERIES?:
A. Tympanic
B. Ophthalmic
C. Internal auditory
D. Superior cerebellar
E. Thalamo-geniculate
Ref. 10 - p. 437

488. THE SUPERIOR SAGITTAL SINUS:
A. Extends from the foramen cecum to the internal occipital protuberance
B. Is located along the free or inferior border of the falx cerebri
C. Decreases in caliber as it proceeds caudally
D. Gives off a number of lateral diverticula called venous lacunae
E. Is joined by the great cerebral vein (Galen) at the anterior border of the tentorium
Ref. 7 - p. 80

489. WHICH OF THE FOLLOWING STATEMENTS CONCERNING THE FORMATION OF THE BRACHIAL PLEXUS ARE INCORRECT?:
A. Formed by the ventral rami of the fifth cervical nerve to the first thoracic nerve
B. Formation of four trunks
C. Separation of each trunk into an anterior and a posterior division
D. Union of divisions to form five cords
E. Derivation from the cords of the principal nerves of distribution
Ref. 11 - p. 80

490. THE LONG THORACIC NERVE:
A. Supplies the serratus anterior muscle
B. Arises from the fifth, sixth, and seventh cervical nerves
C. Supplies the rhomboid muscle
D. May be referred to as Bell's nerve and result in a winged scapula when damaged
E. Arises from the lateral cord
Ref. 11 - p. 81

491. THE LUMBAR PLEXUS:
A. Is formed from the ventral rami of the first three lumbar nerves and part of the fourth lumbar nerve
B. Includes the obturator and femoral nerves
C. Has no connection with the sympathetic trunk
D. Includes the sciatic nerve
E. Gives rise to the pudendal nerve Ref. 11 - p. 456

492. THE CAVERNOUS PLEXUS:
A. Continues as a plexus along the external carotid artery
B. Gives rise to the petrosal nerve
C. Forms the nerve plexus for the vertebral artery
D. Sends fibers to the ciliary ganglion
E. Sends branches to the blood vessels of the hypophysis
Ref. 11 - p. 280

493. THE SENSORY NERVES OF THE DURA MATER ARE DERIVED FROM WHICH OF THE FOLLOWING NERVES?:
A. All three divisions of the trigeminal
B. Vagus
C. Oculomotor
D. Trochlear
E. Glossopharyngeal Ref. 11 - pp. 276-277

494. THE TENTORIUM CEREBELLI:
A. Separates the cerebellar hemispheres
B. Is elevated in the median line
C. Is attached at its circumference to the edges of the grooves for the transverse sinuses
D. Occupies the longitudinal cerebral fissure
E. Separates the cerebellum from the cerebral hemispheres
Ref. 11 - p. 274

495. WHICH OF THE FOLLOWING STATEMENTS MAY BE APPLIED TO THE PROCESS OF AGING OF THE NERVOUS SYSTEM?:
A. A gross atrophy with a disproportionate increase in the size of the ventricles
B. Appearance of calcification in the meninges
C. Atrophy of the pacchionian bodies
D. Cell counts in older individuals indicate an increase in neurons
E. The nucleus may become irregular in shape and disappear
Ref. 9 - p. 35

496. WHICH OF THE FOLLOWING TERMS OR STATEMENTS APPLY TO THE SYMPATHETIC DIVISION OF THE AUTONOMIC NERVOUS SYSTEM?:
A. Preganglionic cell bodies are located within the lateral intermediate gray columns
B. Pelvic splanchnic nerves
C. Stellate ganglion
D. Vagus nerve
E. Ganglion impar Ref. 8 - p. 147

497. WHICH OF THE FOLLOWING TERMS OR STATEMENTS APPLY TO THE PARASYMPATHETIC DIVISION OF THE AUTONOMIC NERVOUS SYSTEM?:
A. White ramus communicans
B. Superior cervical ganglion
C. Craniosacral outflow
D. Thoracico lumbar outflow
E. Vagus nerve Ref. 8 - p. 152

498. STIMULATION OF PARASYMPATHETIC FIBERS:
A. Slows the heart
B. Causes dilation of the pupil
C. Induces sweat secretion
D. Induces piloerection
E. Increases secretion of the lacrimal gland
Ref. 8 - pp. 156-157

499. THE DENERVATION OF SYMPATHETIC FIBER MIGHT RESULT IN WHICH OF THE FOLLOWING?:
A. Increased parotid secretion
B. Ptosis
C. Constriction of the pupil
D. Increased heart rate
E. Increased secretion by the sweat glands
Ref. 8 - pp. 155-157

500. WHICH OF THE FOLLOWING STRUCTURES ARE INNERVATED BY THE PARASYMPATHETIC DIVISION OF THE AUTONOMIC NERVOUS SYSTEM?:
A. Blood vessels of the lower extremity
B. Extensor carpi radalis longus muscle
C. Stomach
D. Salivary glands
E. Palmaris longus muscle Ref. 8 - pp. 154, 156, 159

501. THE NUCLEUS DORSALIS:
A. Is a group of large cells in the lateral part of the anterior column
B. Extends from the last cervical to the second lumbar segment
C. May be referred to as the column of Clarke
D. Is located in the medial part of the base of the posterior column
E. Is not a prominent feature in cross-sections of the thoracic cord
Ref. 12 - p. 176

502. THE FASCICULUS PROPRIUS:
A. Consists of ascending and descending fibers
B. Is primarily concerned with contralateral reflexes
C. Is located within the posterior gray columns
D. Surrounds the gray columns
E. Arises and terminates within the gray substance of the cord
Ref. 12 - p. 174

503. RENSHAW CELLS:
A. Are located on the medial aspect of the posterior columns
B. Excite all types of motor neurons
C. Are supplied by collaterals of the motor cells supplying skeletal muscle
D. Are located in the medial part of the ventral horn of gray matter
E. Are found in the substantia gelatinosa
Ref. 12 - p. 181

504. THE DESCENDING BRANCHES OF THE FIBERS OF THE MEDIAL DIVISION OF THE DORSAL ROOT CONTRIBUTE TO WHICH OF THE FOLLOWING PATHWAYS?:
A. Dorsolateral fasciculus
B. Fasciculus interfascicularis
C. Tract of Lissauer
D. Septomarginal fasciculus
E. Comma tract of Schultz Ref. 12 - pp. 186, 187

505. THE DORSAL SPINOCEREBELLAR TRACT:
A. Begins in the upper lumbar segments
B. Consists of large fibers which take origin from the cells of the nucleus dorsalis
C. Is a well defined bundle of fibers located in the dorsal funiculus
D. Transmits impulses to the cerebellum from the muscles of the trunk and legs
E. Is not a prominent feature of the sections through the thoracic portion of the cord Ref. 12 - p. 188

506. THE VENTRAL SPINOCEREBELLAR TRACT:
A. May be called Gower's tract
B. Consists of fibers which arise from the cells of the posterior gray column of the same and the opposite side
C. Is concerned with the transmission to the cerebellum of afferent impulses from muscles, joints, tendons and skin at a subconscious level
D. May be called the tract of Flechsig
E. Is concerned with conscious proprioception
Ref. 12 - p. 189

507. THE VENTRAL SPINOTHALAMIC TRACT:
A. Is a descending pathway
B. Is assigned crude touch and pressure sense
C. Consists of fibers which take origin from cells in the posterior gray column of the same side
D. Is concerned with subconscious proprioception
E. Terminates within the thalamus Ref. 12 - p. 190

508. THE LATERAL SPINOTHALAMIC TRACT:
A. Is concerned with pain and temperature sensibility
B. Terminates mainly in the ventral posterolateral nucleus of the thalamus
C. Is concerned with crude touch and pressure sense
D. Has neurons of the second order in the dorsal gray columns
E. Has neurons of the first order in the substantia gelatinosa Rolandi
Ref. 6 - p. 88

509. THE FIRST ORDER NEURONS FOR CONSCIOUS PROPRIOCEPTION ARE LOCATED IN THE:
A. Dorsolateral tract of Lissauer
B. Thalamus
C. Nucleus gracilis
D. Nucleus cuneatus
E. Dorsal root ganglia Ref. 6 - p. 90

510. THE FASCICULUS CUNEATUS CARRIES WHICH OF THE FOLLOWING SENSORY MODALITIES?:
A. Pain and temperature
B. Conscious proprioception
C. Subconscious proprioception
D. Discriminative touch
E. Two-point discrimination Ref. 6 - p. 90

511. WHERE ARE SECOND ORDER NEURONS CONCERNED WITH POSITION SENSE, STEREOGNOSIS AND VIBRATORY SENSE LOCATED?:
A. Thalamus
B. Nucleus gracilis
C. Dorsal gray column
D. Dorsal root ganglia
E. Nucleus cuneatus Ref. 6 - p. 90

512. THE SPINOTECTAL TRACT:
A. Arises from cells in the anterior gray column
B. Ascends in the lateral funciulus
C. Terminates in the tectum of the mesencephalon
D. Accompanies the ventral spinothalamic tract
E. Carries reflex connections with other afferent impulses such as auditory and visual Ref. 12 - p. 193

513. WHICH OF THE FOLLOWING DESCENDING FIBER TRACTS ARE LOCATED IN THE ANTERIOR FUNICULUS?:
A. Vestibulospinal
B. Tectospinal
C. Rubrospinal
D. Bulbospinal
E. Septomarginal
Ref. 12 - p. 194

514. THE CORTICOSPINAL TRACTS:
A. Descend through the internal capsule
B. Carry pain fibers
C. Have a role in precise and dexterous voluntary movements
D. Originate in the upper brain stem
E. Descend in the posterior funiculus Ref. 6 - p. 98

515. WHICH OF THE FOLLOWING TRACTS ORIGINATE IN THE MIDBRAIN AND TERMINATE IN THE SPINAL CORD?:
A. Vestibulospinal
B. Reticulospinal
C. Rubrospinal
D. Tectospinal
E. Corticospinal
Ref. 6 - p. 98

516. THE VESTIBULOSPINAL TRACTS:
A. Take origin in the lower brain stem
B. Exert inhibitory influences through alpha motor neurons
C. Have their origin in the vestibular nuclei
D. Exert facilitatory influences through alpha and gamma motor neurons on muscle tone
E. Pass through the internal capsule Ref. 6 - p. 98

517. THE CELLS OF ORIGIN OF THE SENSORY FIBERS OF THE CRANIAL NERVES:
A. Lie outside the cerebrospinal axis
B. Are found within the brain stem
C. Are all bipolar cells
D. Are homologous with sensory cells of dorsal root ganglia
E. Send their axons into the central nervous system
Ref. 12 - p. 202

518. THE DECUSSATION OF THE PYRAMIDS OCCUR:
A. Near the caudal extremity of the medulla oblongata
B. In the internal capsule
C. Above the decussation of the medial lemniscus
D. In the pons
E. In the thoracic region of the spinal cord
Ref. 12 - p. 207

519. INTERNAL ARCUATE FIBERS OF THE MEDULLA OBLONGATA ARISE FROM WHICH OF THE FOLLOWING AREAS?:
A. Gracile and cuneate nuclei
B. Sensory nuclei of the cranial nerves
C. Olivocerebellar fibers
D. Cells of the reticular formation
E. Cells of the lateral cuneate nucleus Ref. 12 - p. 210

520. THE NUCLEUS OF THE TRACTUS SOLITARIUS IS THE NUCLEUS OF RECEPTION OF THE AFFERENT FIBERS FOR WHICH OF THE FOLLOWING CRANIAL NERVES?:
A. Trigeminal
B. Vagus
C. Facial
D. Oculomotor
E. Glossopharyngeal
Ref. 12 - p. 216

521. THE DORSAL MOTOR NUCLEUS OF THE VAGUS:
A. Occupies the ala cinerea of the rhomboid fossa
B. Lies along the medial side of the hypoglossal nucleus
C. Is found in the mesencephalon
D. Is concerned with general visceral efferent fibers
E. Gives rise to efferent fibers of the vagus nerve which innervate smooth muscle and glandular tissue Ref. 12 - p. 216

522. THE NUCLEUS OF THE HYPOGLOSSAL NERVE:
A. Is located in the pons
B. Lies immediately beneath that part of the floor of the fourth ventricle called the trigonum hypoglossi
C. Gives rise to fibers which pass through the reticular formation to emerge at the lateral border of the pyramid
D. Gives origin to motor fibers which supply striated musculature of the pharynx
E. Is medial to the nucleus intercalatus Ref. 12 - p. 216

523. THE INFERIOR CEREBELLAR PEDUNCLE IS COMPOSED OF WHICH OF THE FOLLOWING FASICLES?:
A. Olivocerebellar fibers
B. Ventral spinocerebellar tract
C. Dorsal external arcuate fibers
D. Spinal tract of the trigeminal nerve
E. Dorsal spinocerebellar tract Ref. 12 - p. 213

524. THE NUCLEUS AMBIGUUS:
A. Is located in the upper part of the pons
B. Contains nerve cells which give origin to motor fibers for striated musculature of the pharynx
C. Sends fibers by way of the glossopharyngeal, vagus and accessory nerves
D. Is located in the mesencephalon
E. Aids in the formation of the medial lemniscus
Ref. 12 - p. 216

ANSWER THE FOLLOWING QUESTIONS (T)RUE OR (F)ALSE:

525. The roof of the midbrain is called the lamina quadrigemina.
Ref. 6 - p. 126

526. The sixth cranial nerve emerges in the caudal aspect of the roof of the midbrain. Ref. 6 - p. 126

527. The tegmentum, which comprises the bulk of the brain stem, is located ventral to the ventricular canal. Ref. 6 - p. 126

528. The reticular system is limited to the brain stem.
Ref. 6 - p. 126

529. The dorsal longitudinal fasciculus is located in the periventricular gray matter. Ref. 6 - p. 127

530. The dorsal longitudinal fasciculus is a pathway associated with the autonomic nervous system. Ref. 6 - p. 127

531. The caudal end of the floor of the fourth ventricle with its markings of grooves and elevations has been named calamus scriptorius.
Ref. 8 - p. 172

532. A chemoreceptor function has been attributed to the area postrema.
Ref. 8 - p. 173

533. The ala cinerea marks the location of the dorsal motor nucleus of the vagus nerve. Ref. 8 - p. 173

534. The hypoglossal trigone lies lateral to the ala cinerea.
Ref. 8 - p. 173

535. The restiform body is also called the inferior cerebellar peduncle.
Ref. 8 - p. 174

536. The dorsal external arcuate fibers arise in the lateral portion of the nucleus. Ref. 8 - p. 175

537. The medial lemniscus is composed of fibers arising in nuclei cuneatus and gracilis. Ref. 8 - p. 175

538. The tractus solitarius coordinates movements of the head, eyes and trunk. Ref. 8 - p. 176

539. The medial longitudinal fasciculus is also called the tract of Schutz. Ref. 8 - p. 177

540. The fibers marking the rostral extent of the medulla and crossing in the floor of the fourth ventricle are named striae medullares. Ref. 8 - p. 177

SELECT THE MOST APPROPRIATE ANSWER(S):

541. SECONDARY AND TERTIARY AUDITORY FIBERS PASS THROUGH WHICH OF THE FOLLOWING PATHWAYS?:
A. Dentatorubrothalamic
B. Lateral lemniscus
C. Medial lemniscus
D. Medial longitudinal fasciculi
E. Brachium pontis
Ref. 8 - p. 180

542. VESTIBULAR FIBERS PASS TO THE OCULOMOTOR, TROCHLEAR AND ABDUCENS NUCLEI BY WHICH OF THE FOLLOWING PATHWAYS?:
A. Striae medullares
B. Tractus solitarius
C. Medial longitudinal fasciculus
D. Medial reticulospinal tract
E. Trigeminal lemnisci
Ref. 8 - p. 180

543. THE SPINAL TRACT OF THE TRIGEMINAL NERVE CARRIES WHICH OF THE FOLLOWING SENSORY MODALITIES?:
A. Pain
B. Touch
C. Temperature
D. Pressure
E. Proprioception
Ref. 8 - p. 182

544. THE MAIN SENSORY NUCLEUS OF THE TRIGEMINAL NERVE IS CONCERNED WITH WHICH OF THE FOLLOWING SENSORY MODALITIES?:
A. Pain
B. Touch
C. Temperature
D. Pressure
E. Proprioception
Ref. 8 - p. 182

545. PRIMARY SENSORY NEURONS BEARING PROPRIOCEPTIVE IMPULSES FROM THE MUSCLES OF MASTICATION ARE LOCATED IN WHICH OF THE FOLLOWING AREAS?:
A. Spinal nucleus of the trigeminal
B. Geniculate ganglion
C. Dorsal root ganglion
D. Mesencephalic nucleus of the trigeminal
E. Semilunar ganglion
Ref. 8 - p. 182

546. THE PONTINE NUCLEI GIVE RISE TO FIBERS WHICH CROSS TO THE OPPOSITE SIDE AND FORM LARGE BUNDLES WHICH PASS INTO THE CEREBELLUM BY WHICH OF THE FOLLOWING ROUTES?:
A. Inferior cerebellar peduncle
B. Middle cerebellar peduncle
C. Restiform body
D. Locus ceruleus
E. Brachium pontis — Ref. 8 - p. 182

547. WHICH OF THE FOLLOWING AREAS OF THE BRAIN STEM SHOW PIGMENTATION?:
A. Inferior colliculus
B. Tectum
C. Substantia nigra
D. Locus ceruleus
E. Dorsal paramedian nucleus — Ref. 8 - pp. 182-183

548. WHICH OF THE FOLLOWING CRANIAL NERVE NUCLEI ARE SITUATED NEAR THE MIDLINE AT THE LEVEL OF THE SUPERIOR AND INFERIOR COLLICULI?:
A. Trochlear
B. Facial
C. Abducens
D. Trigeminal
E. Oculomotor
Ref. 8 - p. 186

549. THE SPECIAL VISCERAL EFFERENT COMPONENTS OF MEDULLARY NERVES ALL ARISE FROM WHICH OF THE FOLLOWING NUCLEI?:
A. Nucleus solitarius
B. Nucleus ambiguus
C. Hypoglossal nucleus
D. Olivary nuclear complex
E. Nucleus gracilis — Ref. 9 - p. 139

550. THE DORSAL TEGMENTAL DECUSSATION:
A. Is called the decussation of Forel
B. Is composed of fibers from the red nucleus
C. Is composed of fibers which arise in the superior colliculi
D. Gives rise to fibers which form the tectobulbar and tectospinal tracts
E. Gives rise to the rubrospinal tract — Ref. 12 - p. 231

551. THE FUNCTIONAL COMPONENTS OF A TYPICAL SPINAL NERVE INCLUDE WHICH OF THE FOLLOWING?:
A. Special somatic afferent
B. General somatic efferent
C. General visceral afferent
D. Special visceral afferent
E. General visceral efferent — Ref. 12 - p. 238

552. THERE ARE __________ DISTINCT FUNCTIONAL COMPONENTS INCLUDED IN CRANIAL NERVES (NOT ALL IN EACH NERVE):
A. 4
B. 9
C. 3
D. 7
E. 5
Ref. 12 - p. 240

553. THE SOMATIC EFFERENT COLUMN INCLUDES THE NUCLEI OF THE:
A. Hypoglossal nerve
B. Abducens nerve
C. Trochlear nerve
D. Vagus nerve
E. Accessory nerve
Ref. 12 - p. 242

554. THE SPECIAL VISCERAL EFFERENT COLUMN INCLUDES THE NUCLEI OF THE:
A. Oculomotor nerve
B. Trigeminal nerve
C. Facial nerve
D. Vagus nerve
E. Trochlear nerve
Ref. 12 - p. 245

555. THE GENERAL VISCERAL EFFERENT COLUMN INCLUDES WHICH OF THE FOLLOWING NUCLEI?:
A. Nucleus ambiguus
B. Superior olivary nuclei
C. Dorsal motor nucleus of the vagus
D. Nucleus salivatorius
E. Edinger-Westphal nucleus
Ref. 12 - p. 248

556. THE NUCLEUS SALIVATORIUS INFERIOR SENDS FIBERS BY WAY OF THE__________NERVE TO THE OTIC GANGLION:
A. Vagus
B. Facial
C. Trigeminal
D. Abducens
E. Glossopharyngeal
Ref. 12 - p. 249

557. THE EDINGER-WESTPHAL NUCLEUS CONTAINS PREGANGLIONIC CELL BODIES WHICH GIVE ORIGIN TO EFFERENT FIBERS THAT RUN TO WHICH OF THE FOLLOWING GANGLIA?:
A. Ciliary
B. Submandibular
C. Otic
D. Pterygopalatine
E. Superior cervical
Ref. 12 - p. 249

558. ALL OF THE VISCERAL AFFERENT FIBERS OF THE CRANIAL NERVES, EXCEPT THOSE OF THE FIRST PAIR, ARE CONTAINED IN WHICH OF THE FOLLOWING NERVES?:
A. Facial
B. Trigeminal
C. Glossopharyngeal
D. Auditory
E. Vagus
Ref. 12 - p. 252

559. ALL GENERAL AND SPECIAL VISCERAL AFFERENT FIBERS ENTER THE BRAIN STEM AND TERMINATE IN A COLUMN OF NERVE CELLS KNOWN AS THE:
A. Nucleus ambiguus
B. Nucleus of tractus solitarius
C. Nucleus salivatorius
D. Vestibular nuclei
E. Cochlear nuclei
Ref. 12 - p. 252

560. THE MAIN SENSORY NUCLEUS OF THE TRIGEMINAL NERVE IS LOCATED AT THE LEVEL OF:
A. The superior colliculus
B. Red nucleus
C. Cephalic end of the medulla
D. Middle of the pons
E. Caudal end of the mesencephalon
Ref. 12 - p. 256

561. THE SPECIAL SOMATIC AFFERENT NUCLEI ARE ASSOCIATED WITH THE__________NERVE:
A. Oculomotor
B. Trochlear
C. Facial
D. Stato-acoustic
E. Glossopharyngeal
Ref. 12 - p. 258

562. THE SPIRAL GANGLION OF THE COCHLEA:
A. Is composed of multipolar cells
B. Contains bipolar cells
C. Contains cells which carry special somatic afferent impulses
D. Is composed of special visceral efferent fibers
E. Is concerned with equilibrium
Ref. 12 - p. 258

563. THE OPTIC TRACTS PARTIALLY ENCIRCLE THE CEREBRAL PEDUNCLES AND RUN TO WHICH OF THE FOLLOWING AREAS?:
A. Medial geniculate body
B. Superior colliculus
C. Lateral geniculate body
D. Inferior colliculus
E. Pretectal region
Ref. 12 - p. 266

564. THE PRETECTAL REGION IS THE ZONE OF TRANSITION BETWEEN THE__________AND THE TECTUM:
A. Hippocampus
B. Thalamus
C. Amygdala
D. Cerebellum
E. Septum
Ref. 12 - p. 267

565. THE SUPERIOR OBLIQUE MUSCLE IS INNERVATED BY WHICH OF THE FOLLOWING CRANIAL NERVES?:
A. Abducens
B. Oculomotor
C. Trochlear
D. Trigeminal
E. Facial
Ref. 12 - p. 271

566. THE________, CONSISTING OF AFFERENT TRIGEMINAL ROOT FIBERS WHICH ENTER THE BRAIN STEM AT UPPER PONTINE LEVELS AND DESCEND, OCCUPIES THE REGION WHICH AT SPINAL LEVELS CONSTITUTES THE ZONE OF LISSAUER:
A. Mesencephalic root
B. Main sensory tract of the trigeminal
C. Medial lemniscus
D. Lateral lemniscus
E. Spinal trigeminal tract
Ref. 7 - p. 311

567. THE VISCERAL MOTOR NUCLEUS OF THE SEVENTH CRANIAL NERVE IS KNOWN AS THE:
A. Inferior salivatory nucleus
B. Superior salivatory nucleus
C. Geniculate ganglion
D. Semilunar ganglion
E. Otic ganglion
Ref. 7 - p. 358

568. THE SPECIAL VISCERAL EFFERENT FIBERS OF THE TRIGEMINAL NERVE INNERVATE WHICH OF THE FOLLOWING MUSCLES?:
A. Levator veli palatini
B. Tensor veli palatini
C. Tensor tympani
D. Lateral pterygoid
E. Zygomaticus major — Ref. 7 - p. 364

569. WHICH OF THE FOLLOWING CRANIAL NERVE NUCLEI ARE ASSOCIATED WITH THE FACIAL NERVE?:
A. Edinger-Westphal nucleus
B. Inferior salivatory nucleus
C. Motor nucleus which sends fibers around abducens nucleus
D. Tractus solitarius nucleus
E. Superior salivatory nuclei — Ref. 6 - p. 142

570. THE RETICULAR FORMATION IS THE INTRICATE NEURAL NETWORK WHICH IS ORGANIZED:
A. Into nuclei
B. Into ascending pathways
C. Only within the boundaries of the medulla
D. Below the mesencephalon
E. As descending pathways — Ref. 6 - p. 126

571. THE THALAMUS FORMS ROUGHLY__________PERCENT OF THE DIENCEPHALON:
A. 40
B. 25
C. 70
D. 80
E. 50
Ref. 10 - p. 223

572. THE THALAMUS IS AN ALMOST SOLID BODY OF GRAY MATTER, ONE OF THE LARGEST IN THE BRAIN, BROKEN ONLY BY__________:
A. Medullary laminae
B. Internal capsule
C. Striae medullaris
D. Stria terminalis
E. External capsule
Ref. 10 - p. 223

573. LATERALLY (AND SOMEWHAT VENTRALLY), THE INTERNAL CAPSULE SEPARATES THE THALAMUS FROM WHICH OF THE FOLLOWING?:
A. Lentiform nucleus
B. Caudate nucleus
C. Hypothalamus
D. Globus pallidus
E. Putamen
Ref. 10 - p. 223

574. THE CAUDATE NUCLEUS IS SEPARATED FROM THE THALAMUS BY A SHALLOW BUT WELL-MARKED GROOVE CALLED THE:
A. Claustrum
B. Medullary laminae
C. Sulcus terminalis
D. Extreme capsule
E. Internal capsule
Ref. 10 - p. 223

575. THE INTRALAMINAR NUCLEI FORM A CHAIN IN THE:
A. Internal medullary lamina
B. Midline nuclei
C. Anterior nucleus
D. Metathalamus
E. Epithalamus — Ref. 10 - p. 227

576. THE CENTRUM MEDIANUM BELONGS TO WHICH OF THE FOLLOWING THALAMIC NUCLEAR GROUPS?:
A. Anterior
B. Midline
C. Intralaminar
D. Lateral
E. Posterior
Ref. 12 - p. 294

577. THE__________GROUP OF NUCLEI RECEIVES FIBERS FROM THE MAMMILLOTHALAMIC TRACT AND SENDS FIBERS TO THE CEREBRAL CORTEX IN THE GYRUS CINGULI:
A. Midline
B. Medial
C. Lateral
D. Anterior
E. Posterior
Ref. 12 - p. 294

578. THE SUBTHALAMIC NUCLEUS:
A. Is also called corpus Luysii
B. Includes the habenular trigone
C. Includes the gray matter which lies upon the medial side of the transition zone between the internal capsule and basis peduncle
D. Is situated between the thalamus and the tegmentum of the mesencephalon
E. Includes the stria medullaris
Ref. 12 - p. 301

579. THE EPITHALAMUS INCLUDES WHICH OF THE FOLLOWING?:
A. Pineal body
B. Fasciculus lenticularis
C. Forel's Field H
D. Stria medullaris
E. Ansa lenticularis
Ref. 12 - p. 301

580. WHICH OF THE FOLLOWING STRUCTURES ARE INCLUDED IN THE METATHALAMUS?:
A. Lateral geniculate body
B. Pulvinar
C. Parataenial nucleus
D. Reticular thalamic nucleus
E. Medial geniculate body
Ref. 6 - p. 201

581. WHICH OF THE FOLLOWING STRUCTURES ARE INCLUDED IN THE MIDLINE THALAMIC NUCLEI?:
A. Parafascicular nucleus
B. Reuniens nucleus
C. Paraventricular nucleus
D. Parataenial nucleus
E. Centrum medianum nucleus
Ref. 6 - p. 201

582. THE LATERAL THALAMIC NUCLEAR GROUP INCLUDES WHICH OF THE FOLLOWING STRUCTURES?:
A. Ventral anterior nucleus
B. Ventral posterior nucleus
C. Lateral dorsal nucleus
D. Rhomboid nucleus
E. Central median nucleus
Ref. 6 - p. 201

ANSWER THE FOLLOWING QUESTIONS (T)RUE OR (F)ALSE:

583. The corpus cerebelli is divided by the primary fissure into an anterior and a posterior lobe. Ref. 8 - p. 268

584. The flocculonodular portion is the oldest part of the cerebellum. Ref. 8 - p. 268

585. The thalamus has long been referred to as the head ganglion of the proprioceptive system. Ref. 8 - p. 267

586. The hemispheric extension of the declive is the posterior semilunar lobule. Ref. 8 - p. 269

587. The hemispheric extension of the folium is the superior semilunar lobule. Ref. 8 - p. 269

588. The cerebellar cortex consists of an outer layer of Purkinje cells. Ref. 8 - p. 270

589. The Purkinje cell bodies of the cerebellar cortex are about 75 to 95 μ in diameter. Ref. 8 - p. 270

590. The largest and most laterally placed cerebellar nucleus is the dentate. Ref. 8 - p. 277

591. The most medial of the cerebellar nuclei are the fastigial. Ref. 8 - p. 277

592. The dentate and interpositus nuclei send all their projections out via the superior cerebellar peduncle. Ref. 8 - p. 277

593. The uncinate fasciculus (of Russell) loops around the inferior cerebellar peduncle before entering the juxtarestiform body. Ref. 8 - p. 279

594. The brachium pontis is composed almost entirely of pontocerebellar fibers. Ref. 8 - p. 281

595. The flocculonodular lobe is primarily concerned with vestibulocerebellar fibers. Ref. 8 - p. 282

596. The tectocerebellar tract arises in the tectum and descends in the posterior medullary velum. Ref. 12 - p. 278

597. The superior cerebellar peduncle undergoes a complete decussation beneath the inferior colliculus in the tegmentum of the mesencephalon. Ref. 12 - p. 281

598. The juxtarestiform body consists of the fibers associated with the vestibular system. Ref. 6 - p. 148

599. The cerebellum has an essential role in the coordination of group muscle activities. Ref. 6 - p. 145

600. Classically, the cerebellum is divided into two large bilateral cerebellar hemispheres and the narrow median vermis.
Ref. 6 - p. 145

SELECT THE MOST APPROPRIATE ANSWER(S):

601. THE MOTOR NUCLEUS OF THE TRIGEMINAL NERVE GIVES RISE TO WHICH OF THE FOLLOWING TYPES OF FIBERS?:
A. Special visceral efferent
B. General somatic efferent
C. General visceral efferent
D. General somatic afferent
E. Special somatic afferent Ref. 9 - p. 171

602. THE CELLS OF THE MOTOR NUCLEUS OF THE TRIGEMINAL NERVE SHOW WHICH OF THE FOLLOWING CHARACTERISTICS?:
A. Small
B. Bipolar
C. Large
D. Multipolar
E. Coarse nissl granules. Ref. 9 - p. 171

603. SECTIONING THE RIGHT TRIGEMINAL NERVE ROOT RESULTS IN WHICH OF THE FOLLOWING?:
A. Interferes seriously with chewing
B. Spastic paralysis
C. Deviation of jaw toward the right side
D. Flaccid paralysis
E. Loss of general visceral efferent Ref. 9 - p. 172

604. MOST OF THE CUTANEOUS INNERVATION OF THE HEAD IS MEDIATED BY THE __________ COMPONENT OF THE TRIGEMINAL NERVE:
A. Special visceral efferent
B. General somatic efferent
C. General visceral efferent
D. General somatic afferent
E. Special somatic afferent Ref. 9 - p. 172

605. THE EXTERNAL EAR IS SUPPLIED BY OVERLAPPING CURTANEOUS BRANCHES OF ALL THE FOLLOWING NERVES, <u>EXCEPT</u> FOR THE:
A. Trigeminal
B. Facial
C. Vagus
D. Accessory
E. Glossopharyngeal
Ref. 9 - p. 172

606. THE CELL BODIES OF THE GENERAL SOMATIC AFFERENT, EXTEROCEPTIVE FIBERS OF THE TRIGEMINAL NERVE ARE IN WHICH OF THE FOLLOWING GANGLIA?:
A. Geniculate
B. Gasserian
C. Semilunar
D. Jugular
E. Nodose
Ref. 9 - p. 172

607. AT CERVICAL LEVELS, THE NUCLEUS OF THE SPINAL TRACT OF THE TRIGEMINAL BECOMES INDISTINGUISHABLE FROM WHICH OF THE FOLLOWING?:
A. Lateral corticospinal
B. Ventral spinothalamic
C. Substantia gelatinosa
D. Fasciculus gracilis
E. Dorsal spinocerebellar Ref. 9 - p. 172

608. THE NUCLEUS OF THE SPINAL TRACT OF THE TRIGEMINAL NERVE HAS BEEN DIVIDED INTO WHICH OF THE FOLLOWING SUBDIVISIONS ?:
A. Subnucleus caudalis
B. Subnucleus cephalad
C. Subnucleus rostralis
D. Subnucleus interpolaris
E. Subnucleus posterior
Ref. 9 - p. 172

609. WHICH OF THE FOLLOWING ARE CHARACTERISTIC OF THE CHIEF SENSORY NUCLEUS OF THE TRIGEMINAL NERVE ?:
A. Lies lateral to the root of V
B. Consists of small to medium sized neurons
C. Ovoid or oblong shaped
D. Third order sensory neurons
E. Second order neurons for pain and temperature
Ref. 9 - p. 173

610. THOSE FIBERS IN THE SPINAL TRACT OF V ARE FUNCTIONALLY RELATED TO IMPULSES SET UP BY__________STIMULI:
A. Conscious proprioception
B. Subconscious proprioception
C. Tactile
D. Pain and temperature
E. Pressure Ref. 9 - p. 174

611. TOTAL SECTION OF THE SPINAL TRACT OF V AT THE CAUDAL END OF THE MEDULLA PRODUCES WHICH OF THE FOLLOWING?:
A. Partial anesthesia to pain on the face on the opposite side of the section
B. Complete anesthesia to pain on the face on the side of the section
C. May have small area around the lips still sensitive to pain
D. Complete anesthesia to pain from the region of the ear
E. Loss of proprioception to muscles of mastication
Ref. 9 - p. 174

612. THE NUCLEUS OF THE MESENCEPHALIC ROOT OF THE TRIGEMINAL CONTAINS CELLS OF ORIGIN FOR THE__________FIBERS OF THE V NERVE:
A. Proprioception
B. Pain
C. Temperature
D. Touch
E. Pressure Ref. 9 - p. 177

613. CHARACTERISTICS OF THE NUCLEUS OF THE MESENCEPHALIC ROOT OF THE TRIGEMINAL INCLUDE WHICH OF THE FOLLOWING?:
A. Composed mainly of multipolar cells
B. Contains first order sensory neurons
C. Extends into the medulla
D. May be separated into intermediate, medial and lateral portions
E. Is primarily related to pain and temperature
Ref. 9 - p. 177

614. WHICH OF THE FOLLOWING STATEMENTS APPLY TO THE TRACT OF LISSAUER?:
A. Dorsolateral fasciculus
B. Cells of origin for this tract are located in the geniculate ganglion
C. Axons forming this tract enter the cord through the lateral division of each dorsal root
D. Gives off collaterals to the underlying substantia gelatinosa
E. Contains second order neuronal fibers
Ref. 9 - p. 76

615. WHICH OF THE FOLLOWING ARE CHARACTERISTIC OF THE DORSOLATERAL TRACT?:
A. Carries conscious proprioceptive impulses
B. Present throughout the length of the spinal cord
C. Tract is largest in area of the cervical enlargements
D. Concerned with pain and temperature
E. Ceases at the upper lumbar segment of the spinal cord
Ref. 9 - p. 76

616. THE LATERAL SPINOTHALAMIC TRACT:
A. Proceeds upward to the anterior thalamic nuclei
B. Contains third order sensory neuronal fibers
C. Proceeds upward to the posterolateral ventral nucleus of the thalamus
D. Carries pain and temperature impulses
E. Joins other ascending systems and turns dorsalward at upper cervical levels
Ref. 9 - p. 79

617. WHICH OF THE FOLLOWING STATEMENTS MAY BE APPLIED TO THE SPINOTECTAL TRACT ?:
A. Related to cutaneous pain
B. Arises from the dorsal funicular gray
C. Decussates in the medial lemniscus
D. Decussates in the pons
E. Decussates through the anterior white commissure
Ref. 9 - p. 79

618. WHICH OF THE FOLLOWING STATEMENTS MAY APPLY TO THE VENTRAL SPINOTHALAMIC TRACT ?:
A. Ascends through brain stem levels to terminate in the posterolateral ventral thalamus
B. Becomes incorporated in the medial lemniscus at the level of the pons
C. Carries general tactile sensibility
D. Decussates in the pons
E. Carries conscious proprioceptive impulses
Ref. 9 - p. 85

619. THE NEURONS MEDIATING THE MOST SPECIFIC TYPE OF TACTILE SENSIBILITY PROBABLY HAVE, IN MAN, THE PERIPHERAL TERMINATIONS IN WHICH OF THE FOLLOWING?:
A. Free nerve endings
B. Meissner's corpuscles
C. Merkel's discs
D. Pacinian corpuscle
E. Golgi-Mazzoni corpuscle. Ref. 9 - p. 87

620. WHICH OF THE FOLLOWING CHARACTERISTICS MAY BE APPLIED TO THE FASCICULUS GRACILIS:
A. Ascends in the lateral gray column
B. Terminates in nuclear masses at uppermost cord and lower medulla levels
C. Carries pain and temperature impulses
D. Lies lateral to the fasciculus cuneatus
E. Contains fibers arising from dorsal root ganglia that supply areas innervated by sacral, lumbar and lower thoracic spinal nerves
Ref. 9 - p. 89

621. WHICH OF THE FOLLOWING CHARACTERISTICS MAY BE APPLIED TO THE DORSAL SPINOCEREBELLAR TRACT?:
A. Contralateral pathway for conscious proprioception
B. Ipsilateral pathway for pain and temperature
C. Axons of second order sensory neurons
D. Is concerned with "stretch-evoked" activity
E. The largest myelinated fibers of the dorsal root terminate in the nucleus of Clarke for relay of impulses to the dorsal spinocerebellar tract Ref. 9 - p. 93

622. WHICH OF THE FOLLOWING CHARACTERISTICS MAY BE APPLIED TO THE VENTRAL SPINOCEREBELLAR TRACT?:
A. Enters the cerebellum by way of the restiform body
B. Is both ipsilateral and contralateral
C. Undergoes a partial decussation in the inferior cerebellar commissure
D. Carries pain and temperature impulses
E. Contains axons of first order sensory neurons
Ref. 9 - p. 93

623. THE SPINO-OLIVARY TRACT IS PRIMARILY CONCERNED WITH WHICH OF THE FOLLOWING?:
A. Proprioception
B. Tactile stimulation
C. Pain and temperature
D. Lower motor neurons
E. Upper motor neurons
Ref. 9 - p. 93

624. PROPRIOCEPTIVE IMPULSES IN MUSCLES, TENDONS AND JOINTS ARE RELAYED TO WHICH OF THE FOLLOWING AREAS?:
A. Cerebellum
B. Lateral vestibular nucleus
C. Hypothalamus
D. Inferior vestibular nucleus
E. Cingulate gyrus Ref. 9 - p. 95

625. THE RUBROSPINAL TRACT IS PRIMARILY CONCERNED WITH WHICH OF THE FOLLOWING?:
A. Pain and temperature
B. Tactile stimulation
C. Extrapyramidal functions
D. Auditory functions
E. Visual functions Ref. 9 - p. 99

626. THE RUBROSPINAL TRACTS CROSS THE MIDLINE IN WHICH OF THE FOLLOWING?:
A. Ventral tegmental decussation
B. Dorsal tegmental decussation
C. Decussation of the pyramids
D. Internal arcuate fibers
E. Inferior cerebellar commissure Ref. 9 - p. 99

627. WHICH OF THE FOLLOWING ARE CHARACTERISTIC OF THE RUBROSPINAL TRACT?:
A. Enters the spinal cord ventral to the ventral corticospinal tract
B. Sends many fibers to the reticular region of the brain stem
C. Many fibers discharge directly to ventral horn motor neurons
D. Rubrospinal fibers cross the midline in the dorsal tegmental decussation
E. Concerned with autonomic impulses Ref. 9 - p. 99

628. WHICH OF THE FOLLOWING ARE CHARACTERISTIC OF THE TECTOSPINAL TRACT?:
A. Contains both medial and lateral bundles
B. Cells of origin are located in the superior colliculus
C. Is concerned with auditory reflexes
D. Is concerned with extrapyramidal discharge
E. Is also called the uncinate fasciculus
Ref. 9 - p. 102

629. THE UNCINATE FASCICULUS ARISES FROM:
A. Superior vestibular nucleus
B. Red nuclei
C. Tegmental nuclei
D. Nucleus fastigii
E. Reticular nuclei Ref. 9 - p. 102

630. WHICH OF THE FOLLOWING ARE CHARACTERISTIC OF THE MEDIAL VESTIBULOSPINAL TRACT?:
A. Arises from the medial, lateral and inferior vestibular nuclei
B. Descends to cord levels ventral to each medial tectospinal tract
C. The fibers end around motor neurons that supply lower extremity musculature
D. Is often termed medial longitudinal fasciculus at spinal cord levels
E. Ends at sacral levels Ref. 9 - p. 104

ANSWER THE FOLLOWING QUESTIONS (T)RUE OR (F)ALSE:

631. The olivospinal tract is part of a system for coordinating upper extremity and head movements. Ref. 9 - p. 104

632. The lateral reticulospinal tract sends some fibers to the cells of the intermediolateral column of the upper thoracic levels. Ref. 9 - p. 104

633. The ventral reticulospinal tract contains some fibers which belong to the temperature-regulating mechanism of the nervous system. Ref. 9 - p. 105

SELECT THE MOST APPROPRIATE ANSWER(S):

634. DORSIFLEXION OF THE GREAT TOE RESULTS IN WHICH OF THESE TESTS?:
A. Hoffmann's reflex
B. Chaddock's sign
C. Oppenheim's sign
D. Gordon's sign
E. Philippe's sign
Ref. 9 - p. 107

635. WHICH OF THE FOLLOWING CHARACTERISTICS ARE TRUE FOR THE SEPTOMARGINAL TRACT?:
A. Concerned with the reception of pain and temperature impulses
B. Is a descending pathway
C. Concerned with the reception of tactile impulses
D. Is found in the lateral funiculus
E. Is found in the dorsal funiculus Ref. 9 - p. 107

636. THE PROPRIUS BUNDLES SURROUND THE GRAY OF THE SPINAL CORD EVERYWHERE, EXCEPT IN THE REGION OF:
A. Corticospinal tract
B. Lissauer's tract
C. Dorsolateral tract
D. Lateral spinothalamic tract
E. Ventral spinothalamic tract Ref. 9 - p. 108

ANSWER THE FOLLOWING QUESTIONS (T)RUE OR (F)ALSE:

637. The caudal limit of the medulla oblongata is limited by the lower border of the foramen magnum. Ref. 9 - p. 112

638. The central canal of the spinal cord ceases at the upper cervical levels. Ref. 9 - p. 112

639. The widest part of the fourth ventricle is at the transition from medulla to spinal cord. Ref. 9 - p. 112

640. The ventricular system of the brain is completely lined with ependyma. Ref. 9 - p. 112

641. The ala cinerea is medial to the hypoglossal trigone. Ref. 9 - p. 114

642. The abducens nerve emerges in line with the hypoglossal nerve at the transition from the medulla oblongata to the pons.
Ref. 9 - p. 115

643. The nucleus of Roller may be termed the parahypoglossal gray.
Ref. 9 - p. 132

644. The special visceral efferent components of medullar nerves arise from the dorsal motor nucleus. Ref. 9 - p. 139

645. General visceral efferent components of the vagus nerve arise from the nucleus ambiguus. Ref. 9 - p. 139

646. The Purkinje cells are the efferent neurons of the cerebellar cortex.
Ref. 9 - p. 193

647. The granular layer is the outer region of the cerebellar cortex.
Ref. 9 - p. 193

648. Stellate cells of the cerebellum are found in the molecular layer.
Ref. 9 - p. 193

649. Golgi cells are located in the granular layer of the cerebellum.
Ref. 9 - p. 195

650. The mossy fibers and the climbing fibers are the afferents to the cerebellar cortex. Ref. 9 - p. 195

SELECT THE MOST APPROPRIATE ANSWER(S):

651. THE ________ NUCLEUS IS OFTEN TERMED THE ROOF NUCLEI OR NUCLEUS TECTI:
A. Dentate
B. Globus
C. Emboliform
D. Fastigial
E. Mammillary
Ref. 9 - p. 198

652. WHICH OF THE FOLLOWING ARE NOT FOUND IN THE INFERIOR CEREBELLAR PEDUNCLE ?:
A. Dorsal spinocerebellar tract
B. Dorsal superficial arcuate fibers
C. Olivocerebellar bundles
D. Dentatorubro fibers
E. Ventral spinocerebellar tract Ref. 9 - p. 200

653. THE DORSAL SPINOCEREBELLAR TRACT ARISES FROM WHICH OF THE FOLLOWING?:
A. Dorsolateral tract of Lissauer
B. Substantia gelatinosa
C. Intermediolateral cell column
D. Clarke's column
E. Anterior horn cells Ref. 9 - p. 200

654. THE STRIAE MEDULLARES ARE FORMED FROM WHICH OF THE FOLLOWING?:
A. Secondary cochlear fibers
B. Arcuato cerebellar fibers
C. Fibers of Piccolomini
D. Secondary pain and temperature fibers
E. Tactile fibers Ref. 9 - p. 202

655. THE MAJOR COMPONENTS OF THE MIDDLE CEREBELLAR PEDUNCLE INCLUDE WHICH OF THE FOLLOWING?:
A. Pontocerebellar bundle
B. Cerebellotegmental fibers
C. Dentatothalamic fibers
D. Dorsal spinocerebellar tract
E. Nucleocerebellar tract Ref. 9 - p. 206

656. THE TECTOCEREBELLAR FIBERS ARE LARGELY FROM:
A. Superior colliculus
B. Red nucleus
C. Basis pedunculi
D. Substantia nigra
E. Inferior colliculus
Ref. 9 - p. 211

657. THE TUBER AND FOLIUM VERMIS PROBABLY RECEIVE WHICH OF THE FOLLOWING FIBERS?:
A. Tectocerebellar
B. Olivocerebellar
C. Pontocerebellar
D. Dorsal spinocerebellar
E. External arcuate
Ref. 9 - p. 211

658. THE BEST-KNOWN CONNECTIONS OF THE BIVENTRAL LOBULE AND THE TONSILLA INCLUDE WHICH OF THE FOLLOWING FIBERS?:
A. Dorsal spinocerebellar
B. Reticulocerebellar
C. Olivocerebellar
D. Pontocerebellar
E. Tectocerebellar
Ref. 9 - p. 212

659. FIBERS FROM THE FLOCCULUS PROJECT TO WHICH OF THE FOLLOWING NUCLEI?:
A. Dentate
B. Oculomotor
C. Trigeminal
D. Hypoglossal
E. Spinal accessory
Ref. 9 - p. 212

660. THE LARGEST AFFERENT SYSTEM TO THE SUPERIOR COLLICULUS INCLUDES WHICH OF THE FOLLOWING TRACTS?:
A. Internal corticotectal
B. Corticomesencephalic
C. Reticulotectal
D. Olivotectal
E. Internal arcuate
Ref. 9 - p. 229

661. THE MIDBRAIN TEGMENTUM CONTAINS WHICH OF THE FOLLOWING BUNDLES?:
A. Basis pedunculi
B. Medial lemniscus
C. Lateral lemniscus
D. Medial longitudinal fasciculus
E. Dorsal spinocerebellar tract Ref. 9 - p. 252

ANSWER THE FOLLOWING QUESTIONS (T)RUE OR (F)ALSE:

662. The decussation of the superior cerebellar peduncles lies at superior collicular levels. Ref. 9 - p. 257

663. There are four commissures that particularly characterize the tegmental area of the midbrain. Ref. 9 - p. 257

664. The dorsal tegmental decussation lies at inferior collicular levels. Ref. 9 - p. 257

SELECT THE MOST APPROPRIATE ANSWER(S):

665. THE MOST ROSTRAL OF THE MIDBRAIN COMMISSURES INCLUDES WHICH OF THE FOLLOWING?:
A. Supramammillary
B. Postmammillary
C. Commissure of Forel
D. Decussation of brachia conjunctiva
E. Dorsal tegmental decussation Ref. 9 - p. 259

666. THE MOST PROMINENT NUCLEAR MASS OF THE BASAL PART OF THE MIDBRAIN INCLUDES WHICH OF THE FOLLOWING?:
A. Superior colliculus
B. Inferior colliculus
C. Substantia nigra
D. Red nucleus
E. Trochlear nucleus
Ref. 9 - p. 260

667. THE HYPOTHALAMIC SULCUS OF HIS IS REGARDED AS THE PROBABLE FORWARD CONTINUATION OF THE:
A. Tectum
B. Tegmentum
C. Basis pedunculi
D. Sulcus limitans
E. Medial lemniscus
Ref. 9 - p. 266

668. THE EPITHALAMUS INCLUDES ALL OF THE FOLLOWING, <u>EXCEPT</u> THE:
A. Pineal organ
B. Habenular commissure
C. Ependymal part of the tela choroidea
D. Part of the posterior commissure
E. Anterior commissure Ref. 9 - p. 267

669. THE NUCLEUS OF DARKSCHEWITSCH IS SOMETIMES TERMED THE VENTRAL NUCLEUS OF THE:
A. Anterior commissure
B. Posterior commissure
C. Thalamus
D. Hypothalamus
E. Mesencephalon
Ref. 9 - p. 268

670. THE LARGEST AND BEST-KNOWN DISCHARGE PATH FROM EACH HABENULA IS THE:
A. Habenulopeduncular tract
B. Fasciculus retroflexus of Meynert
C. Tectohabenular
D. Habenulotectal
E. Stria terminalis Ref. 9 - p. 272

671. THE NUCLEUS VENTRALIS POSTEROLATERALIS IS THE THALAMIC REGION OF TERMINATION FOR WHICH OF THE FOLLOWING TRACTS?:
A. Lateral spinothalamic
B. Stria terminalis
C. Stria medullaris
D. Ventral spinothalamic
E. Fornix
Ref. 9 - p. 288

672. THE ANTERIOR VENTRAL NUCLEUS OF THE THALAMUS RECEIVES IMPULSES FROM THE GLOBUS PALLIDUS BY WAY OF THE:
A. Stria medullaris
B. Stria terminalis
C. Medial forebrain bundle
D. Thalamic fasciculus
E. Habenulopeduncular tract
Ref. 9 - p. 294

673. THE MAJOR NUCLEAR MASSES OF THE ________ THALAMUS ARE THE ZONA INCERTA WITH THE ASSOCIATED NUCLEUS OF THE FIELD OF FOREL:
A. Dorsal
B. Ventral
C. Anterior
D. Posterior
E. Medial
Ref. 9 - p. 307

674. THE ZONA INCERTA IS LOCATED WHERE?:
A. Midbrain
B. Epithalamus
C. Metathalamus
D. Immediately ventral to the dorsal thalamus
E. Below the plane of the hypothalamic sulcus
Ref. 9 - p. 307

675. WHICH OF THE FOLLOWING CHARACTERISTICS DO NOT APPLY TO THE SUBTHALAMIC NUCLEI?:
A. Lies along the lateral border of the internal capsule
B. Poor blood supply
C. Contains all spindle-shaped cells
D. Has the approximate shape of a biconvex lens
E. Is clearly evident in the 3 cm human embryo
Ref. 9 - p. 308

ANSWER THE FOLLOWING QUESTIONS (T)RUE OR (F)ALSE:

676. The subthalamic nucleus apparently serves as a relay in an extra-pyramidal system. Ref. 9 - p. 309

677. The arcuate nucleus of the hypothalamus may be called the infundibular nucleus. Ref. 9 - p. 310

678. The lateral mammillary nucleus makes up the main mass of the mammillary bodies. Ref. 9 - p. 310

679. The fornix is surrounded for part of the way by the perifornical nucleus. Ref. 9 - p. 312

680. The hypothalamohypophyseal tract constitutes the major nerve supply to the pars nervosa. Ref. 9 - p. 325

SELECT THE MOST APPROPRIATE ANSWER(S):

681. THE __________ IS A THIN SHEET OF BRAIN SUBSTANCE MARKING THE ROSTRAL END OF THE EMBRYONIC BRAIN:
A. Anterior medullary velum
B. Lamina terminalis
C. Corpus callosum
D. Hippocampus
E. Septum pelludicum — Ref. 9 - p. 343

682. THE FORNICATE LOBE INCLUDES ALL OF THE FOLLOWING, EXCEPT FOR THE:
A. Uncus
B. Cingulate
C. Hippocampal gyrus
D. Isthmus
E. Corpus callosum
Ref. 9 - p. 349

683. THE MAJOR EFFERENT DISCHARGE SYSTEM OF THE LENTICULAR COMPLEX INCLUDES WHICH OF THE FOLLOWING?:
A. Stria terminalis
B. Fornix
C. Lenticular fasciculus
D. Subthalamic fasciculus
E. Pallidohypothalamic fasciculus — Ref. 9 - p. 372

684. IN THE MIDBRAIN THE LENTICULAR FASCICULUS ENDS PRIMARILY IN WHICH OF THE FOLLOWING?:
A. Nucleus of Darkschewitsch
B. Zona incerta
C. Interstitial nucleus of the medial longitudinal fasciculus
D. Superior colliculus
E. Deep tegmental gray — Ref. 9 - p. 375

685. THE __________ LIES BETWEEN THE EXTERNAL AND EXTREME CAPSULES:
A. Putamen
B. Globus pallidus
C. Claustrum
D. Substantia nigra
E. Red nucleus
Ref. 9 - p. 388

ANSWER THE FOLLOWING QUESTIONS (T)RUE OR (F)ALSE:

686. The average thickness of the cortex is approximately 2.5 mm.
Ref. 9 - p. 410

687. The motor area is thickest of all the cortex.
Ref. 9 - p. 410

688. The visual cortex is about 4.5 mm in thickness.
Ref. 9 - p. 410

689. The weight of a newborn male brain is approximately 400 gm.
Ref. 9 - p. 410

690. The olfactory ventricle is usually present in adult olfactory bulbs.
Ref. 9 - p. 414

691. The rostral portions of the cingulate gyrus have agranular cortex. Ref. 9 - p. 473

692. Area 4 is thought to be bounded rostrally by a suppressor area. Ref. 9 - p. 480

693. Area 4 is characterized cytoarchitecturally by a modification of layers I and II. Ref. 9 - p. 480

694. The upper extremity area of the motor cortex, and particularly the shoulder and neck regions, are better differentiated in the newborn than the lower extremity region. Ref. 9 - p. 482

695. The face area of the motor cortex is the most dorsal portion. Ref. 9 - p. 482

696. Area 6 lacks the giant pyramidal cells characteristic of area 4. Ref. 9 - p. 493

697. A supplementary motor area exists at the base of the precentral and postcentral gyrus. Ref. 9 - p. 493

698. Area 22 is concerned with auditory receptivity. Ref. 9 - p. 514

699. Rhythmic speech is said to have bilateral representation in the parietal cortex. Ref. 9 - p. 514

700. The insula is supplied from its external surface by branches of the middle cerebral artery. Ref. 9 - p. 558

FOR EACH OF THE FOLLOWING MULTIPLE CHOICE QUESTIONS, SELECT THE MOST APPROPRIATE ANSWER(S):

701. A STIMULUS ACTS ON AN EXCITABLE CELL TO BRING ABOUT A TRANSIENT DEPOLARIZATION BY:
A. Decreasing the permeability of the cell membrane to Na^+
B. Increasing the permeability of the cell membrane to Na^+ or to Na^+ and K^+
C. Retaining the resting permeability of the cell membrane to Na^+
D. Decreasing the permeability of the cell membrane to K^+
E. None of these Ref. 17 - p. 27

702. AN ACTION POTENTIAL IS DEFINED AS:
A. Depolarization followed by repolarization
B. The spread of a wave over the membrane of the entire cell
C. The voltage change accompanying a nerve impulse
D. Propagation of the impulse from the stimulus site to adjacent regions of the membrane
E. Spontaneous recovery of the nerve following depolarization
Ref. 17 - p. 27

703. THE FOLLOWING ITEM IS OUT OF ORDER IN THE SEQUENCE OF EVENTS CONSTITUTING THE IMPULSES OF A SIMPLE REFLEX ARC:
A. Stimulus initiates impulses in nerve endings
B. Impulses propagated over afferent nerve fibers
C. Efferent fibers traverse ventral root of spinal cord
D. Impulses initiated in motor neuron
E. Impulses activate contraction of muscle cells
Ref. 12 - p. 27

704. THE SIZE OF THE RESTING POTENTIAL ACROSS NERVE AND MUSCLE MEMBRANES DEPENDS LARGELY ON THE:
A. Relative permeability of the membrane to sodium and potassium ions
B. Size of the nerve fiber or muscle cell
C. Ratio of the permeability of potassium to that of sodium
D. Internal sodium concentration
E. Internal potassium concentration Ref. 17 - p. 29

705. THE PASSAGE OF AN ACTION POTENTIAL CONSISTS OF ALL THE FOLLOWING SEQUENCE OF CHANGES, EXCEPT:
A. Latency prior to beginning of action potential
B. A rapid decrease of membrane potential toward zero
C. A brief reversal of the membrane potential so that the inside becomes positive to the outside
D. A slow reversal of membrane potential to the resting level
E. A second overshoot of the membrane potential
Ref. 17 - p. 29

706. THE THRESHOLD OF AN ACTION POTENTIAL IS DEFINED AS:
A. Maximal response of a muscle fiber
B. Minimal stimulus strength to evoke a propagating action potential
C. Maximal stimulus strength to evoke a propagating action potential
D. Minimal response of a muscle fiber
E. Fixed conduction speed of a given nerve fiber
Ref. 17 - p. 29

707. AN ACTION POTENTIAL HAS THE FOLLOWING CHARACTERISTIC:
A. Maximal response to a threshold stimulus
B. Increased response to increased stimulus following threshold intensity
C. Slight response to a threshold stimulus
D. No response to a threshold stimulus
E. None of these Ref. 17 - p. 39

708. THE PRINCIPLE OF A STRENGTH-DURATION CURVE IS THAT:
A. The threshold current strength for a prolonged stimulus is less than for a shorter stimulus
B. The threshold current strength for a prolonged stimulus is more than for a shorter stimulus
C. The threshold current strength for a prolonged stimulus is the same as for a shorter stimulus
D. Latency is directly proportional to the length of the stimulus
E. The threshold current strength is equal to the chronaxie
Ref. 17 - pp. 39-40

709. SALTATORY CONDUCTION IN NERVE FIBER IS:
A. An even conduction flow along the nerve axon
B. Nerve conduction of an unmyelinated fiber
C. Propagation of the nerve impulse from Node of Ranvier to Node of Ranvier
D. Decrease in conduction time related to decreased myelin
E. The effect of a saline solution application to the nerve at the time of stimulus Ref. 17 - p. 47

710. INVESTIGATIONS OF NERVE CONDUCTION SPEED INDICATE THAT:
A. In unmyelinated fibers, speed is proportional to the diameter
B. Distance between nodes is not a factor in myelinated fibers
C. Speed is minimized by a thick myelin sheath
D. In myelinated fibers, speed is directly proportional to diameter
E. Resistance of the axoplasm is proportional to the cross sectional area of the fiber Ref. 17 - p. 48

711. WHICH OF THE FOLLOWING PHYSICAL FACTORS HAS NO INFLUENCE ON SPEED OF THE NERVE IMPULSE?:
A. Temperature
B. Resistivity of the cell plasm
C. Amount of threshold voltage
D. Size of the membrane capacitor
E. Extent of the increase in sodium permeability
Ref. 17 - p. 48

712. THE ACTIVITY OF A STIMULATED BUNDLE OF NERVE FIBERS IS CALLED:
A. Negative after potential
B. Positive after potential
C. Transmembrane voltage
D. Generator potential
E. Compound action potential Ref. 17 - pp. 73-74

713. WHEN A NERVE TRUNK IS EXCITED BY A MAXIMAL STIMULUS, THE RESULTING RECORD SHOWS THAT:
A. Fibers with the lowest threshold conduct most rapidly
B. All fibers conduct at the same velocity
C. Unmyelinated fibers conduct the most rapidly
D. The smallest fibers conduct the most rapidly
E. Fibers with the highest threshold stimulus conduct most rapidly
Ref. 17 - pp. 75-77

714. IN THE RECORD OF A COMPOUND ACTION POTENTIAL OF A CAT'S SAPHENOUS NERVE, THE FIRST AND HIGHEST ELEVATION IS THE RESULT OF RESPONSE OF:
A. A fibers
B. B fibers
C. C fibers
D. Postganglionic sympathetic fibers
E. Unmyelinated afferent fibers Ref. 17 - pp. 76-78

715. WHICH OF THE FOLLOWING GROUPS OF NERVE AXONS ARE CLASSIFIED AS TYPE B?:
A. Myelinated, somatic, afferent and efferent fibers
B. Myelinated efferent, preganglionic, autonomic fibers
C. Efferent postganglionic sympathetic axons
D. Small unmyelinated afferent axons
E. A and D Ref. 17 - p. 81

716. LARGE AFFERENT NERVE FIBERS (12-21 u) ARE CHARACTERIZED BY:
A. Representation in all somatic nerve trunks
B. Being unmyelinated
C. Being entirely motor fibers
D. Being confined to muscle nerves
E. Belonging to sympathetic nerves Ref. 17 - p. 83

717. WHEN AN AXON IS SEVERED, ALL BUT ONE OF THE FOLLOWING CHANGES OCCUR:
A. Wallerian degeneration
B. Alteration of myelin
C. Few or no alterations in the neuron cell body
D. Proliferation of Schwann cells
E. Dissolution of the axis cylinder Ref. 17 - p. 84

718. THE MOST RAPIDLY CONDUCTING NERVE FIBERS IN THE SPINAL CORD CONDUCT AT RATES UP TO:
A. 70 m. per second
B. 30 m. per second
C. 60 m. per second
D. 40 m. per second
E. 120 m. per second Ref. 17 - p. 93

719. IN GENERAL, NERVE FIBERS IN THE CENTRAL NERVOUS SYSTEM AS COMPARED WITH PERIPHERAL NERVE FIBERS HAVE:
A. Lower refractory periods
B. Greater diameter-velocity relation
C. Greater velocity-threshold relation
D. The same properties of conduction
E. Shorter refractory periods Ref. 17 - p. 93

720. THE CRITICAL FIRST EVENT IN NATURAL IMPULSE INITIATION IN THE BODY IS:
A. Decreased sodium permeability
B. Membrane depolarization
C. Subthreshold polarization
D. Electrical threshold stimulus
E. Membrane hyperpolarization Ref. 17 - p. 95

721. THE TERMINAL AFFERENT ENDINGS WHICH UNDERGO DEPOLARIZATION IN RESPONSE TO SPECIFIC KINDS OF STIMULI ARE CALLED:
A. Nerve ganglia
B. Sensory nerve cell bodies
C. Receptors
D. Efferent neurons
E. Sensory presynaptic neurons Ref. 17 - p. 95

722. THE GENERATOR OR RECEPTOR POTENTIAL IS THE MEMBRANE POTENTIAL DECREASE PRODUCED IN THE TERMINAL NERVE ENDINGS IN RESPONSE TO STIMULI. IDENTIFY ITS CHARACTERISTICS FROM THE FOLLOWING LIST:

1. All or none
2. Graded and stationary
3. Independent of stimulus intensity
4. Diminished rapidly with distance along fiber
5. Self propagating

A. 2 and 4 D. 4 and 5
B. 1 E. 1 and 3
C. 3 Ref. 17 - p. 96

723. HIGH-THRESHOLD RECEPTORS WHOSE EXCITATION GIVES RISE TO PAIN SENSATIONS ARE:
A. Interoceptors D. Tonic receptors
B. Nociceptors E. None of these
C. Phasic receptors Ref. 17 - p. 97

724. ENCAPSULATED PACINIAN CORPUSCLES IN THE MESENTERY ARE SELECTIVELY SENSITIVE TO:
A. Heat
B. Touch
C. Movement
D. Rapid compression of the capsule
E. Cold Ref. 17 - p. 97

725. THE PROCESS OF ADAPTATION IS DEFINED AS:
A. Increase in magnitude of the generator potential during sustained stimulation
B. Increase in conduction rate during sustained stimulation
C. Decrease in magnitude of the generator potential during sustained stimulation
D. Decrease in conduction rate upon sustained stimulation
E. Decrease in magnitude of the generator potential during brief stimulation Ref. 17 - p. 101

726. AN EXAMPLE OF A PHASIC RECEPTOR IS A:
A. Pacinian corpuscle
B. Muscle stretch receptor
C. Tendon stretch receptor
D. Pressoreceptor in carotid sinus
E. Certain thermal receptors Ref. 17 - p. 102

727. IN THE RECEPTOR IMPULSE THE DEPOLARIZATION OF THE GENERATOR REGION RESULTS IN:
A. Blocking of the receptor impulse
B. Triggering of repetitive discharge of all - or none spikes
C. Elicitation of only a steady depolarization of the immediate region
D. Propagation along the fiber by the local circuit mechanism
E. B and D Ref. 17 - p. 105

728. THE ABSOLUTE REFRACTORY PERIOD OF A NERVE IS THE PERIOD DURING WHICH:
A. A second shock of increased resting threshold intensity will excite
B. A second shock of decreased resting threshold will excite
C. A second stimulus of any type is completely ineffective
D. An intense steady stimulus will excite
E. A weaker steady stimulus will excite
Ref. 17 - p. 108

729. INHIBITORY IMPULSES APPEAR TO INFLUENCE THE STRETCH RECEPTOR MEMBRANE BY ALL THE FOLLOWING, EXCEPT:
A. Increasing selectively permeability of K^+ and Cl^- ions
B. Selectively decreasing permeability to K^+ and Cl^- ions
C. Reducing sensitivity of the receptor to its adequate stimulus
D. Increasing permeability of the membrane to ions close to true electrochemical equilibum
E. By liberating a chemical agent which selectively alters the ionic permeability of the dendritic membrane
Ref. 17 - p. 112

730. EVENTS IN A SPINAL MOTOR NEURON LEADING TO CONTRACTION OF THE MUSCLE FIBERS IT INNERVATES ARE AS FOLLOWS, EXCEPT:
A. A stimulus initiates a volley of impulses
B. The impulse is conducted along the axon to the muscle's motor end plate
C. Na^+ is liberated from the axon terminals
D. A threshold depolarization of the muscle fiber is induced followed by a self propagating impulse
E. A brief phasic contraction of the muscle fiber - a twitch
Ref. 17 - p. 114

731. ALL OF THE FOLLOWING FACTS ABOUT MOTOR UNITS ARE TRUE, EXCEPT:
A. Number of motor axons innervating a muscle are a small fraction of the total number of muscle fibers
B. A motor axon innervates 1 - 300 muscle fibers
C. Are defined as motoneurons and the muscle fibers each innervates
D. The contractile response to one motoneuron is a twitch contraction of all the fibers it innervates
E. The smallest unit of muscular activity is the contraction of a single motor unit Ref. 17 - p. 115

732. SEQUENCE OF EVENTS OF NEUROMUSCULAR TRANSMISSION CONSISTS OF ALL, EXCEPT:
A. Crossing of a low resistance connection between the axoplasm and the sarcoplasm
B. Depolarization of the naked nerve terminal causes release of ACL
C. ACL diffuses across the gap between nerve ending and end plate
D. Permeability of end-plate membrane to Na^+ and K^+ increased
E. ACL receptor complex quickly destroyed by enzyme, acetylcholinesterase Ref. 17 - pp. 133-134

733. DIRECTLY INVOLVED IN THE RELEASE OF ACL AT THE NEUROMUSCULAR JUNCTION IS:
A. Magnesium
B. Calcium
C. Phosphorus
D. Sodium
E. All of these
Ref. 17 - pp. 135-136

734. THE ACTION OF THE AGENT, CURARE, ON NEUROMUSCULAR TRANSMISSION IS TO:
A. Compete with acetylcholinesterase for receptor sites
B. Cause release of all ACL at receptor site
C. Increase end-plate potential above muscle membrane threshold
D. Block the nerve action potential
E. Block transmission by reducing the end-plate potential below threshold of the muscle membrane Ref. 17 - p. 136

735. SYNAPSES HAVE ALL THE FOLLOWING PROPERTIES, EXCEPT:
A. Unidirectional conduction
B. Repetitive discharge
C. Susceptibility to asphyxia
D. Constant and faithful transmission of frequencies of presynaptic volleys
E. Synaptic delay Ref. 17 - p. 154

736. WHEN A GROUP I AFFERENT VOLLEY OF IMPULSES IS DIRECTED INTO THE SPINAL CORD, THE FOLLOWING CHANGES OCCUR:
A. A transmitter is liberated at the homonymous synapses
B. Permeability to all ions is increased
C. Short circuits occur in some cells because of many active synaptic knobs
D. All of the above
E. None of the above Ref. 17 - p. 179

737. RESULTS OF THE CROSSED EXTENSION REFLEX ARE:
A. Withdrawal of the stimulated limb
B. Withdrawal of the non-stimulated limb
C. Contraction of contralateral flexor muscles
D. Contraction of contralateral extensor muscles
E. Both A and D Ref. 17 - p. 182

738. THE TENDON JERK IS CHARACTERIZED BY:
A. Short latency
B. Presence of afterdischarge
C. Enhancement by strong stimulation
D. Enhancement by Group I afferent volleys in nerves to antagnostic muscles
E. Inhibitory input arising only from synergist muscles
Ref. 17 - pp. 184-185

739. ADEQUATE STIMULUS FOR THE REFLEX MECHANISM OF THE TENDON JERK IS:
A. Electrical stimulation
B. Painful pinch
C. Heat stimulation
D. Stretch of the muscle
E. All of these Ref. 17 - p. 186

740. MUSCLE TONE IS DEFINED AS:
A. Ability of a muscle to contract
B. Resting length of the muscle
C. Resistance of a muscle to passive stretch
D. Ability of a muscle to relax
E. The number of active muscle fibers Ref. 17 - p. 188

741. RECEPTORS PARTICULARLY INVOLVED WITH POSTURAL REFLEXES ARE:
A. Free nerve endings
B. Pacinian corpuscles
C. Encapsulated skin receptors
D. Kraus end organs
E. Muscle spindles Ref. 17 - p. 189

742. MUSCLE SPINDLES INCLUDE ALL THE FOLLOWING STRUCTURES, EXCEPT:
A. Intrafusal fibers
B. Extrafusal fibers
C. Nuclear bag
D. Myotube region
E. Annulospiral nerve endings Ref. 17 - p. 189

743. ALL STRETCH-SENSITIVE UNITS HAVE THE FOLLOWING PROPERTIES IN COMMON, EXCEPT:
A. Response to stretch with a regular discharge of impulses
B. In a limited range of applied tensions, firing rate is approximately directly proportional to the log of the applied muscle tension
C. As stimulus intensity increases, the number of units responding increases
D. Each receptor fires at a frequency determined by the excess of stimulus over threshold of the receptor
E. All have low thresholds to muscle stretch
Ref. 17 - pp. 191-193

744. THE "CLASP KNIFE" REFLEX IN A DECEREBRATE PREPARATION HAS THE FOLLOWING CHARACTERISTIC:
A. Resistance to forcible extension of rigid limb
B. Decrease in resistance throughout initial part of bending
C. Increase in resistance to stretch at midpoint of range of motion
D. Muscle first resists flexion, then relaxes
Ref. 17 - p. 195

745. THE EXCITIBILITY (MEMBRANE POTENTIAL) OF A NEURON AT ANY POINT IN TIME DEPENDS UPON:
A. Strength of the stimuli applied
B. Length of the stimuli applied
C. Number of incoming excitatory impulses
D. Balance of incoming inhibitory and facilitatory influences
E. A and C Ref. 17 - p. 198

746. INVESTIGATION HAS SHOWN THAT CONTRACTILE TENSION OF MUSCLE IS PRODUCED BY:
A. Alpha motor fibers to extrafusal muscle fibers
B. Gamma fibers to extrafusal muscle fibers
C. Gamma fibers to intrafusal muscle fibers
D. Alpha fibers to intrafusal muscle fibers
E. Both Alpha and Gamma fibers Ref. 17 - p. 199

747. GAMMA EFFERENT FIBERS ARE DISTRIBUTED EXCLUSIVELY TO:
A. Extrafusal muscle fibers
B. Smooth muscle fibers
C. Cardiac muscle fibers
D. Tendons
E. Spindle intrafusal fibers Ref. 17 - pp. 199-200

748. AFFERENT DISCHARGE OF THE MUSCLE SPINDLE IS DETERMINED BY:
A. Varying degrees of stretch
B. Number of fusimotor impulses reaching the spindle
C. Contraction of extrafusal muscle fibers
D. Stimulation of cutaneous receptors
E. All of these Ref. 17 - pp. 200-203

749. SPINAL SHOCK IN MAN IS CHARACTERIZED BY ALL THE FOLLOWING, EXCEPT:
A. Follows sectioning of the spinal cord
B. Exaggeration of all reflexes
C. Suppression of all reflexes
D. Post-transectional areflexia
E. Temporary alteration of reflexes Ref. 17 - p. 207

750. CHARACTERISTICS OF A PATIENT WITH SPINAL CORD TRANSECTION MAY CONSIST OF:
A. Flexion reflexes and Babinski sign
B. Mass withdrawal reflexes
C. Extensor reflexes and supporting reactions
D. Autonomic reflexes
E. All of these Ref. 17 - p. 208

751. DEPRESSION OF REFLEXES IN SPINAL SHOCK IS BROUGHT ABOUT BY:
A. Injury to posterior spinal roots
B. Injury to anterior spinal roots
C. Loss of converging descending pathways which summate with segmental afferent input
D. Loss of segmental afferent input
E. Loss of anterior horn cells Ref. 17 - p. 209

752. HYPERACTIVE TENDON REFLEXES AFTER RECOVERY FROM SPINAL SHOCK REPRESENT:
A. Heightened fusimotor discharge
B. Increased Alpha motoneuron excitability
C. Increased muscle spindle sensitivity
D. Strong inhibitory affect of descending pathways on Gamma efferent neurons
E. Recovery of sensory neurons Ref. 17 - p. 210

753. WHICH OF THE FOLLOWING STATEMENTS ARE TRUE IN RELATION TO SENSORY INPUT?:

1. The brain influences gamma neurons which govern sensitivity of muscle spindles
2. Fusimotor control has motor rather than sensory significance
3. Many brain structures exert control on the first synapse in ascending systems
4. The influence of descending pathways on ascending pathways tends to be excitatory

A. 1 only
B. 2 and 3
C. 1, 2 and 3
D. 3 and 4
E. All of the statements Ref. 17 - p. 213

754. CHARACTERISTICS OF THE RETICULOSPINAL TRACTS ARE:
A. Threshold stimulation near the midline tends to inhibit extensor tonus
B. Threshold stimulation near the midline tends to inhibit flexor contraction
C. Lateral stimulation tends to facilitate decerebrate rigidity and inhibit flexion
D. A and B
E. A and C Ref. 17 - p. 217

755. IT HAS BEEN SHOWN THAT BRAIN STEM DESCENDING PATHWAYS FUNCTION AS FOLLOWS:
A. Vestibular neurons facilitate myotatic reflexes of extensor muscles
B. Vestibular neurons inhibit myotatic reflexes of extensor muscles
C. Vestibular neurons do not influence myotatic reflexes of extensor muscles
D. Reticular neurons inhibit myotatic reflexes of extensor muscles
E. Reticular neurons do not influence myotatic reflexes
Ref. 17 - p. 218

756. POSTROTATIONAL NYSTAGMUS IS:
A. The same as tonic labyrinthine reactions
B. Initiated in the eyes
C. Initiated by the semicircular canals
D. Identical with local static reactions
E. A segmental static reaction Ref. 17 - p. 218

757. SEGMENTAL STATIC REACTIONS ARE THE RESULT OF:
A. Influence of spinal segments of one level on those of another level
B. Only exteroceptive stimuli
C. A spinal reflex at one segmental level
D. Labyrinthine reflexes
E. Brainstem influence on the spinal cord
Ref. 17 - p. 219

758. TONIC NECK REFLEXES ELICITED BY ROTATION OF THE JAW TO THE RIGHT FOLLOWING DESTRUCTION OF BOTH LABRYINTHS ARE SOURCES OF STIMULATION FOR THE FOLLOWING STATIC REACTIONS:
A. Increase in extensor posture of both limbs on the right
B. Relaxation of the limbs on the left
C. Relaxation of both right limbs and increase extensor posture of both left limbs
D. Increase in flexor posture of both right limbs and of extensor posture in both left limbs
E. A and B Ref. 17 - p. 220

759. LOCAL STATIC REACTIONS IN LOW DECEREBRATE ANIMALS:
A. Are involved primarily with stance
B. Consist mainly of crossed extension reflexes
C. Result from afferents of one muscle acting upon fellow muscles of the same segment on the opposite side
D. Consist of neck and labryinthine reflexes
E. Arise from position of the head in space
Ref. 17 - p. 219

760. IN A LOW DECEREBRATE ANIMAL, THE TONIC LABYRINTHINE REACTIONS:
A. Depend on the semicircular canals alone
B. Result from tonic neck mechanisms
C. Are probably mediated by the otoliths
D. Result in flexion of the animals extremities when he lies supine
E. None of these Ref. 17 - p. 220

761. IF THE LABYRINTHS AND NECK MUSCLES ARE DENERVATED AND THE ANIMAL IS DROPPED, RIGHTING CAN STILL OCCUR BECAUSE OF THE:
A. Labyrinthine righting reflexes
B. Optical righting reflexes
C. Neck righting reflexes
D. Placing reactions
E. Tonic neck reflexes Ref. 17 - p. 221

762. WHICH OF THE FOLLOWING IS NOT TRUE REGARDING THE LABYRINTH?:
A. Plane of each anterior semicircular canal is parallel to the anterior canal of the opposite side
B. Membranous canals lie within the bony labyrinth
C. The ampulla is at one end of each canal
D. The cupola responds to hydrostatic forces
E. In the ampulla are crista containing hair cell receptors
Ref. 17 - p. 222

763. NYSTAGMUS NORMALLY RESULTS FROM RAPID ROTATION OF THE BODY. IT CAN BE DEFINED AS:
A. Crossing of the eyes
B. Turning of both eyes lateralward
C. Alternate movement of the eyes
D. A squint of one eye
E. Turning of one eye upward and the other downward
Ref. 17 - p. 223

764. EVIDENCE CONCERNING FUNCTION OF THE SACCULE GIVES THE CURRENT BELIEF THAT IT:
A. Is an essential part of the vestibular mechanism
B. Is associated with tilting movements
C. Responds best to rotatory movements
D. Is associated with rapid vibrational movements
E. Is associated with reception of slow vibrational stimuli
Ref. 17 - p. 225

765. THE TYPICAL AUTONOMIC REFLEX CHAIN:
A. Involves only one neuron
B. Involves motor innervation to striated skeletal muscle
C. Involves motor innervation of smooth muscle
D. Has neuronal cell bodies located exclusively in the spinal cord
E. Has neuronal cell bodies located in the dorsal root ganglion
Ref. 17 - p. 227

766. PARASYMPATHETIC AUTONOMIC OUTFLOW ORIGINATES IN THE:
A. Anterior horn of the cervical spinal cord
B. Thoracolumbar spinal cord
C. Cerebral cortex
D. Nuclei of cranial nerves
E. Prevertebral parasympathetic plexuses
Ref. 17 - p. 228

767. THE FUNCTION OF PARASYMPATHETIC INNERVATION TO THE LACRIMAL GLANDS IS:
A. Vasoconstriction
B. Vasodilation and secretion
C. Vasoconstriction and secretion
D. Vasodilation and inhibition of secretion
E. Transmission of pain impulses Ref. 17 - p. 228

768. FUNCTION OF SYMPATHETIC INNERVATION OF THE EYE CONSISTS OF ALL, EXCEPT:
A. Pupillary constriction
B. Pupillary dilation
C. Vasoconstriction
D. Elevation of the lid
E. Accommodation for far vision Ref. 17 - p. 229

769. THE FUNCTION OF PARASYMPATHETIC INNERVATION OF THE HEART IS:
A. Cardiac acceleration
B. Coronary dilation
C. Cardiac deceleration
D. A and B
E. No function
Ref. 17 - p. 229

770. SYMPATHETIC INNERVATION OF THE VISCERA RESULTS IN ALL BUT:
A. Vasoconstriction of blood vessels
B. Inhibition of peristalsis
C. Secretion in adrenal medulla
D. Glycogenolysis in the liver
E. Stimulation of peristalsis
Ref. 17 - p. 231

771. ALL THE FOLLOWING ORGANS RECEIVE ONLY SYMPATHETIC INNERVATION, EXCEPT:
A. Adrenal medulla
B. Sweat glands
C. Pilomotor muscles
D. Lungs
E. Many vascular beds of skin Ref. 17 - p. 231

772. SECTION OF AUTONOMIC NERVES USUALLY RESULTS IN:
A. Degeneration of smooth muscle innervated
B. Alteration of form of organs
C. Alteration of physiological function
D. Autonomous continuation of function
E. B and C Ref. 17 - p. 232

773. ALL THE FOLLOWING STATEMENTS ARE TRUE ABOUT NEUROMUSCULAR TRANSMISSION IN THE AUTONOMIC NERVOUS SYSTEM, EXCEPT:
A. Is associated with increments of contraction
B. Persists after nerve fibers have repolarized
C. Resulting tension curve is prolonged
D. Transmitter is destroyed rapidly and its action is brief
E. Destruction of the transmitter is slow
Ref. 17 - p. 233

774. ALL OF THE FOLLOWING ARE CHOLINERGIC FIBERS, EXCEPT:
A. Sympathetic postganglionic fibers
B. Somatic motor fibers
C. Autonomic preganglionic fibers
D. Parasympathetic postganglionic fibers
E. Sympathetic postganglionic fibers to sweat glands
Ref. 17 - p. 233

775. IF THE BRAIN STEM IS TRANSECTED AT THE INTERCOLLICULAR LEVEL ALL OF THE FOLLOWING EXIST IMMEDIATELY, EXCEPT:
A. Lack of temperature regulation
B. Depression of all autonomic reflexes
C. Absence of sweating
D. Hypotension
E. Retention of medullary vasomotor regulation
Ref. 17 - pp. 238-239

776. SECTIONING OF THE PYRAMIDS IN MONKEYS RESULTS IN:
A. Definite flaccidity of muscles
B. Definite spasticity
C. Presence of abdominal reflexes
D. Presence of cremasteric reflexes
E. Absence of Babinski sign Ref. 17 - p. 275

777. FUNCTIONS OF THE CEREBELLUM INCLUDE THE FOLLOWING:
A. Regulation of skilled movements
B. Influence on tactual, visual and auditory impulses
C. Regulation of visceral activities
D. Regulation of posture and tonus
E. All of these Ref. 17 - p. 289

778. EXTEROCEPTORS HAVE THE FUNCTION OF:
A. Giving information about movement
B. Giving information on changes in the immediate external environment
C. Transmitting impulses from visceral organs
D. Giving information about remote environment
E. Controlling equilibrium Ref. 17 - p. 304

779. THE "DOCTRINE OF SPECIFIC NERVE ENERGIES" HAS A BASIC PRINCIPLE:
A. A sense organ can be stimulated by other than its adequate stimulus
B. Sensory response is of the same subjective response regardless of the kind of stimulus
C. Modality of sensation depends upon what end organ is stimulated
D. Modality of sensation depends upon what nerve fiber is stimulated
E. All of these Ref. 17 - p. 304

780. WEDDELL'S IDEA OF THE BASIS OF SENSATION IS THAT:
A. Spatial patterns of fibers and temporal patterns determine quality of sensation
B. All cutaneous organs respond to specific types of stimulus
C. All sensations can be localized but with varying accuracy
D. Noxious stimuli release a chemical substance in the skin which stimulates end organs
E. None of these Ref. 17 - p. 305

781. SMALL UNMYELINATED C NERVE FIBERS HAVE THE FOLLOWING CHARACTERISTICS:
A. Subserve only pain sensation
B. Respond only to heavy pressure on the skin
C. Do not respond to temperature change
D. Respond only to one form of energy
E. Respond to several forms of energy Ref. 17 - p. 307

782. THE FOLLOWING STATEMENT APPLIES TO TEMPERATURE SENSES:
A. Existence of separate temperature senses for cold and warmth
B. A single temperature sense for hot and cold
C. Absence of a microscopic anatomic receptor specificity disproves functional specificity
D. Most, though not all, impulses underlying thermal sensation are conducted in unmyelinated fibers
E. None of these Ref. 17 - pp. 307-310

783. ALL THE FOLLOWING FACTS ABOUT THE SENSORY MECHANISM FOR PAIN ARE TRUE, EXCEPT:
A. Sensory end organs exist in virtually all tissues of the body
B. Three kinds of pain have been recognized - superficial, deep and visceral
C. Pain endings exhibit to a marked degree the phenomenon of adequate stimulus
D. Pain endings are not specialized to react to a single form of energy
E. Function of pain sense is protective Ref. 17 - p. 311

784. DEEP SENSIBILITY (KINESTHESIS OR PROPRIOCEPTION) IS SUBSERVED BY ALL THE FOLLOWING SENSE ORGANS, EXCEPT:
A. Muscle spindles
B. Golgi tendon organs
C. Joint Pacinian corpuscles
D. Quickly adapting joint capsule receptors
E. Free nerve endings Ref. 17 - p. 313

785. VIBRATORY SENSIBILITY IMPULSES:
A. Are conducted in the anterolateral columns of the spinal cord
B. Are conducted in the posterior columns of the spinal cord
C. Are radically affected by cerebral lesions
D. Have no clinical diagnostic value
E. All of these Ref. 17 - p. 314

786. STEREOGNOSIS HAS THE FOLLOWING CHARACTERISTICS:
A. Appreciation of the forms of three dimensional objects of palpation without vision
B. Involves the synthesis of several modalities of somatic sensation
C. Is extremely affected by lesions of the posterior parietal lobe
D. All of the above Ref. 17 - p. 316

787. DERMATOMES ARE IMPORTANT TO CLINICAL NEUROLOGY BECAUSE:
A. They are identical with peripheral nerve fields
B. They are definite skin areas with no overlapping
C. They indicate the area of skin supplied with afferent fibers of a single posterior root
D. Areas of anesthesia always result from sectioning a single posterior root
E. Sizes of dermatomes are the same for all sensory modalities
Ref. 17 - p. 319

788. THE FOLLOWING EVIDENCE EXISTS FOR THE PRESENCE OF A FAST AND SLOW SYSTEM OF PAIN FIBERS:
A. Pain sensation from a brief stimulus is often experienced as two peaks of pain
B. Interval between pulses is greater when stimuli are applied to the distal end of an extremity than when applied to the proximal end
C. Interval in B is compatible with the difference between C and delta rates of conduction
D. All of the above
E. None of the above Ref. 17 - p. 321

789. IMPULSES CONDUCTED IN THE ANTEROLATERAL TRACTS OF THE SPINAL CORD SUBSERVE ALL OF THE FOLLOWING, <u>EXCEPT</u>:
A. Pain
B. Warmth
C. Cold
D. Muscle, tendon, joint sensibility
E. Touch Ref. 17 - p. 322

790. IMPULSES CONDUCTED IN THE POSTERIOR WHITE COLUMNS OF THE SPINAL CORD CONSIST OF ALL OF THE FOLLOWING, <u>EXCEPT</u>:
A. Two point discrimination
B. Pain
C. Appreciation of vibration
D. Stereognosis
E. Passive movement Ref. 17 - p. 325

791. PAIN AND TEMPERATURE SENSIBILITY OF THE FACE PASS EXCLUSIVELY BY WAY OF THE:
A. Spinal nucleus of the trigeminal nerve
B. Main sensory nucleus of the trigeminal
C. Mesencephalic nucleus of the trigeminal
D. Abducens nucleus of nerve VI
E. Facial nucleus of nerve VII Ref. 17 - p. 325

792. ALL OF THE SENSORY PATHWAYS HAVE A SYNAPSE IN THE THALAMUS, EXCEPT:
A. Touch
B. Pressure
C. Proprioception
D. Olfaction
E. Vision
Ref. 17 - p. 326

793. STUDIES OF TOPOGRAPHIC ORGANIZATION OF THE THALAMUS HAVE REVEALED THAT:
A. Impulses from the face are received in the arcuate nucleus
B. Impulses from the body are received in the nucleus ventralis posterolateralis
C. Body surface representation is projected onto the thalamus
D. A point on the body surface is projected to a specific point on the thalamus
E. All of these
Ref. 17 - pp. 327-328

794. EVOKED POTENTIALS OF SENSORY CORTEX IN RESPONSE TO STIMULATION OF BODY SURFACE HAVE SHOWN THAT:
A. Parts of ipsilateral body surfaces are presented in orderly sequence
B. Parts of contralateral body surfaces are presented in unorganized fashion
C. Parts of contralateral body surfaces are presented in orderly sequence
D. Stimulation of the face elicits only contralateral responses
E. All of the above
Ref. 17 - p. 328

795. ABLATION OF THE CEREBRAL CORTEX IMMEDIATELY IN FRONT OF AND BEHIND THE POSTCENTRAL GYRUS PRODUCES THE FOLLOWING RESULTS:

1. No degeneration in thalamic nuclei
2. Retrograde degeneration in the classic relay thalamic nuclei
3. Retrograde degeneration in thalamic nuclei other than the classic relay group
4. All of these

A. 1
B. 2 and 3
C. 4
D. 3
Ref. 17 - pp. 330-331

796. ABLATION OF THE PARIETAL LOBE IN PRIMATES RESULTS IN ALL OF THE FOLLOWING, EXCEPT:
A. Reduction of ability to discriminate roughness and weight
B. Less effect on ability to discriminate weight and roughness than when postcentral gyrus is ablated
C. Permanent discriminative effects
D. Recovery of reduced discriminative results
E. Reduction in ability to discriminate geometric forms
Ref. 17 - pp. 334-335

797. CORTICAL LESIONS IN MAN USUALLY PRODUCE:
A. Permanent anesthesia for modalities of sensation
B. Transient anesthesia for modalities of sensation
C. Persisting subcortical damage
D. Decrease in threshold for eliciting sensation
E. Simultaneous recovery of pain, pressure and temperature responses
Ref. 17 - pp. 335-336

798. CORTICAL LESIONS HAVE THE FOLLOWING EFFECT ON PAIN:
A. Increase the pain
B. Abolish the pain
C. Affect pain only slightly and temporarily
D. Have more effect than peripheral stimulus
E. Result in the "thalamic syndrome" Ref. 17 - pp. 337-338

799. PRIMARY HYPERALGESIA HAS ALL OF THE FOLLOWING CHARACTERISTICS, EXCEPT:
A. Pain threshold is lowered
B. Pain response is intense
C. Is accompanied by vasodilation
D. Extends beyond the area of damage
E. Never is present for more than 48 hours
Ref. 17 - pp. 346-348

800. DEEP PAIN HAS ALL THE FOLLOWING CHARACTERISTICS, EXCEPT:
A. Originates in muscles, tendons and joints
B. Impulses usually traverse muscle branches of mixed nerves
C. Quality is dull or aching
D. Impulses usually traverse sympathetic nerve fibers
E. Shows the phenomena of referred pain
Ref. 17 - pp. 350-353

801. ADEQUATE PAIN STIMULI FOR VISCERAL AFFERENTS CONSIST OF ALL, EXCEPT:
A. Sudden distension against resistance
B. Spasms or strong contractions
C. Traction on the mesentery
D. Chemical irritants
E. Mechanical stimulation Ref. 17 - p. 353

802. VISCERAL PAIN FIBERS ARE CONDUCTED MAINLY VIA THE:
A. Parasympathetic nerves
B. Somatic nerves
C. Sympathetic nerves
D. All of these Ref. 17 - p. 353

803. THE CONVERGENCE-FACILITATION THEORY OF REFERRED PAIN STATES THAT:
A. Some visceral afferents converge with some cutaneous pain afferents upon the same neuron in the pain pathway
B. The system of fibers is organized topographically
C. The topographic organization provides the dermatomal reference
D. All of A, B and C
E. Afferent impulses from the viscera facilitate normal somatic pain impulses from the skin Ref. 17 - p. 357

804. ANIMALS WITH THEIR PERIPHERAL TASTE NERVES SECTIONED:
A. Select foodstuffs to correct dietary deficiencies
B. If adrenalectomized, selectively drink saline solution
C. If vitamin deficient, will selectively eat foods providing the deficient vitamin
D. Tend to eat and drink indiscriminately Ref. 17 - p. 368

805. THE AFFERENT LIMBS OF THE FOLLOWING REFLEXES ARE FOUND IN SYMPATHETIC NERVES:
A. Cardiac reflexes
B. Aortic reflexes
C. Hering-Breuer reflexes
D. All of these
E. None of these
Ref. 17 - p. 372

806. THE FOLLOWING SIMILARITIES EXIST BETWEEN SOMATIC AND SYMPATHETIC AFFERENTS, EXCEPT FOR:
A. Active fibers are of A delta or C size
B. Fibers of both project to the cerebral cortex
C. Special cortical areas are devoted to both
D. Special thalamic areas are devoted to both
E. Both C and D Ref. 17 - p. 373

807. HUNGER CONTRACTIONS DISAPPEAR IN ALL BUT ONE OF THE FOLLOWING SITUATIONS:
A. Ingestion of food
B. Strong emotional states
C. Sleep
D. Vagotomy
E. Smoking Ref. 17 - p. 375

808. THE FOLLOWING ARE TRUE IN REGARD TO MOTION SICKNESS:
A. Occurs when speed or direction of motion is repeatedly varied
B. Responsible receptors are in the vestibular apparatus
C. Can be induced by uniform continuous movement in one direction
D. All of the above
E. Only A, B and D Ref. 17 - p. 377

809. CHANGES OF ATMOSPHERIC PRESSURE MAY PRESENT PROBLEMS OF AIR PRESSURE IN THE MIDDLE EAR. WHICH OF THE FOLLOWING STATEMENTS ARE TRUE?:
A. Pain results from negative pressures of 60-80 mm Hg.
B. At pressures of 60-80 mm Hg. the ear drum may rupture
C. Pressure differences may produce traumatic inflammation of the middle ear
D. All of the above
E. A and C Ref. 17 - p. 382

810. THE PITCH OF THE SIMPLEST SOUND WAVE IS LARGELY DETERMINED BY:
A. Both amplitude and frequency
B. Its frequency
C. Perceptual response to the intensity
D. Unique wave form of each sound
E. All of these Ref. 17 - p. 382

811. SOUND WAVES IN THE EAR REACH THE ORGAN OF CORTI BY THE FOLLOWING:
A. Physiologic or ossicular route
B. Air route
C. Osseous route
D. All the these
E. None of these Ref. 17 - pp. 392-393

812. DEAFNESS IS GREATLY BENEFITED BY HEARING AIDS IN:
A. Nerve deafness
B. Conduction deafness
C. Central deafness
D. All of these
E. None of these Ref. 17 - p. 393

813. FUNCTIONS OF NEURONS ARE AFFECTED BY WHICH OF THE FOLLOWING?:
A. Size of cell bodies
B. Length and numbers of dendrites
C. Numbers of presynaptic terminals
D. All of the above
E. None of the above Ref. 26 - p. 66

814. THE EXCITATORY TRANSMITTER AT A SYNAPSE IS BELIEVED TO BE STORED IN THE:
A. Synaptic cleft
B. Mitochondria
C. Synaptic gutter
D. Synaptic vesicles
E. Postsynaptic neuron Ref. 26 - p. 67

815. AN IMPORTANT SYNAPTIC TRANSMITTER SUBSTANCE AT PERIPHERAL SYMPATHETIC NERVE ENDINGS IS:
A. Neostigmine
B. Acetylcholine
C. Norepinephrine
D. Gamma aminobutyric acid
E. None of these Ref. 26 - p. 68

816. SIMULTANEOUS EXCITATION OF SUCCESSIVELY GREATER NUMBERS OF EXCITATORY PRESYNAPTIC TERMINALS RESULTS IN:
A. Temporal summation
B. Higher threshold for excitation
C. Decrease in postsynaptic potential
D. Spatial summation
E. A and C Ref. 26 - p. 69

817. POSTULATED TO BE AN INHIBITORY TRANSMITTER IS:
A. Acetylcholine
B. Gamma aminobutyric acid
C. Aminoacid glycine
D. All of the above
E. Only B and C Ref. 26 - p. 72

818. THE POSTULATED MECHANISM OF POSTSYNAPTIC INHIBITION IS THAT THE TRANSMITTER CAUSES:
A. A decrease in the permeability of the neuronal membrane to potassium and chloride ions
B. An increase in the permeability of the neuronal membrane to potassium and chloride ions
C. An increase in permeability of the neuronal membrane to sodium ions
D. A decrease in the permeability of the neuronal membrane to sodium ions
E. B and C Ref. 26 - p. 71

819. THE BELL-MAGENDIE LAW STATES THAT:
A. Conduction through synapses may be transmitted in both directions
B. Synaptic delay of approximately 0.5 milliseconds always occurs
C. Conduction through synapses goes only from presynaptic neurons to successive neurons
D. Upon repetitive stimulation of presynaptic terminals the number of postsynaptic discharges becomes progressively fewer
E. Rapidly successive discharges from the same presynaptic terminal always summate Ref. 26 - p. 72

820. SYNAPTIC TRANSMISSION MAY BE GREATLY DECREASED BY WHICH OF THE FOLLOWING INFLUENCES?:
A. Alkalosis
B. Acidosis
C. Hypoxia
D. Anesthetics
E. All except A
Ref. 26 - p. 73

821. ALL OF THE FOLLOWING ARE CHARACTERISTIC OF THE NEUROMUSCULAR JUNCTION, EXCEPT:
A. Mitochondria
B. Excitatory transmitter acetylcholine
C. Large aggregates of cholinesterase
D. Synthesis of epinephrine
E. An end plate potential 3-4x that is required to stimulate the muscle fiber Ref. 26 - p. 75

822. ALL OF THE FOLLOWING SUBSTANCES STIMULATE MUSCLE ACTION, EXCEPT:
A. Methacholine
B. Carbachol
C. Curare
D. Nicotine
E. Acetylcholine
Ref. 26 - p. 75

823. THE NEUROGENIC SYSTEM FOR REGULATION OF RESPIRATION CONSISTS OF ALL THE FOLLOWING, EXCEPT THE:
A. Medullary respiratory center
B. Pneumotaxic area
C. Thalamic center
D. Apneustic area
E. Vagal and glossopharyngeal nerves Ref. 26 - pp. 494-495

824. THE HERING-BREUER REFLEXES:
A. Prevent overdistention of the lungs
B. Occur only during inspiration
C. Do not affect respiratory rhythm
D. Act only to inhibit inspiration
E. Have no effect on tidal volume Ref. 26 - p. 496

825. THE AUTONOMIC NERVOUS SYSTEM:
A. Controls skeletal muscle
B. Is entirely a sensory system
C. Is both a motor and sensory system
D. Controls smooth muscle and glands
E. Controls diaphragm contraction Ref. 26 - p. 541

826. THE WITHDRAWAL REFLEX IS PROTECTIVE AND:
A. Consists of a number of neurons
B. Consists of only two neurons
C. Is a muscle stretch reflex
D. Prevents sudden changes in muscle length
E. Consists of a sensory nerve fiber which synapses directly with a motor neuron Ref. 26 - p. 543

827. AFTER AN ANIMAL'S BRAIN IS REMOVED, SPINAL CORD FUNCTIONS MAY ALLOW ALL OF THE FOLLOWING, EXCEPT:
A. Ability to stand
B. Reflex emptying of the bladder
C. When suspended in a sling, to make walking movements
D. Scratching in response to skin stimulation
E. Control of equilibrium Ref. 26 - p. 543

828. THE CEREBRAL CORTEX IS ABSOLUTELY ESSENTIAL FOR:
A. Perception of sensation
B. Ability to think
C. Coordinate turning of the head
D. Interpretation of sensations
E. Emotional patterns of anger and excitement
Ref. 26 - pp. 543-544

829. WHEN SIGNALS OF INCREASING STRENGTH ARE TRANSMITTED BY INCREASING THE FREQUENCY OF NERVE IMPULSES IN EACH FIBER, THE PROCESS IS CALLED:
A. Spatial summation
B. Temporal summation
C. Temporal pattern
D. Facilitation
E. Convergence
Ref. 26 - p. 547

830. A SUBTHRESHOLD STIMULUS OF NEURONS:
A. Fails to elicit excitement
B. Causes minimal excitement
C. Is identical with a threshold stimulus
D. Makes the neuron less excitable
E. Does not summate to result in a threshold stimulus
Ref. 26 - p. 549

831. WHEN A NEURON IS MADE MORE EXCITABLE BUT DOES NOT DISCHARGE, THE PROCESS IS CALLED:
A. Threshold stimulation
B. Convergence
C. Summation
D. Facilitation
E. None of these
Ref. 26 - p. 549

832. CENTRIFUGAL NERVE FIBERS CARRY IMPULSES FROM:
A. Skin toward the central nervous system
B. The thalamus to the cerebral cortex
C. Motor areas of the cortex downward
D. Spinal cord to midbrain
E. Muscles to the spinal cord
Ref. 26 - p. 552

833. REVERBERATING CIRCUITS MAY HAVE ANY OF THE FOLLOWING CHARACTERISTICS, EXCEPT:
A. A single neuron with a collateral fiber back to its own dendrites
B. Occurrence in only a single neuronal pool
C. Several neurons in a feedback circuit
D. Many parallel fibers with wide diffusion of terminal fibers
E. Occurrence in a circuit of neuronal pools
Ref. 26 - p. 554

834. ONE OF THE MOST IMPORTANT FACTORS WHICH MIGHT SHORTEN THE DURATION OF A REVERBERATING DISCHARGE IS:
A. Increase in the number of neurons in the pathway
B. Decrease in the number of neurons in the pathway
C. Increased facilitation of the neuronal pool
D. Decreased inhibition of the neuronal pool
E. Rapidity of synaptic fatigue
Ref. 26 - p. 555

835. VOLTAGE IN A GENERATOR POTENTIAL OF A PACINIAN CORPUSCLE:
A. Decreases rapidly when stimulus is first applied
B. Increases more rapidly the higher the stimulus strength
C. Can be almost as high as an action potential
D. None of these
Ref. 26 - p. 559

836. ADAPTATION OF SENSORY RECEPTORS:
A. Is characteristic of only some sensory receptors
B. Occurs at the same rate in all receptors
C. Is characteristic of all sensory receptors
D. Is the result of the same method in all sensory receptors
E. Is not influenced by the structure of the receptor
Ref. 26 - p. 560

837. ALL OF THE FOLLOWING ARE POORLY ADAPTING RECEPTORS, EXCEPT:
A. Pacinian corpuscles
B. Joint capsule receptors
C. Muscle spindles
D. Sound receptors of the ear
E. Pain receptors
Ref. 26 - p. 561

838. THE FOLLOWING ARE CHARACTERISTICS OF PHASIC RECEPTORS, EXCEPT THAT THEY:
A. React strongly while a change is taking place
B. Transmit impulses related to movement
C. Are important for maintenance of body balance
D. Adapt rapidly
E. Adapt slowly Ref. 26 - p. 561

839. TONIC RECEPTORS:
A. Adapt rapidly
B. Detect rate of movement
C. Give information relating to body position
D. Are called rate receptors
E. Are found in Pacinian corpuscles Ref. 26 - p. 561

840. ALL OF THE FOLLOWING ARE SPECIAL SENSES, EXCEPT:
A. Sight
B. Pain
C. Hearing
D. Smell
E. Taste
Ref. 26 - p. 565

841. PROPRIOCEPTIVE SENSATIONS INCLUDE:
A. Kinesthetic
B. Exteroceptive
C. Visceral
D. Deep pressure
E. Vibration
Ref. 26 - p. 565

842. TACTILE RECEPTORS INCLUDE ALL THE FOLLOWING, EXCEPT:
A. Free nerve endings
B. Meissner's corpuscles
C. Golgi tendon organs
D. Hair end-organs
E. Ruffini end-organs Ref. 26 - p. 566

843. KINESTHETIC RECEPTORS INCLUDE ALL THE FOLLOWING, EXCEPT:
A. Ruffini end-organs
B. Golgi tendon receptors
C. Pacinian corpuscles
D. Free nerve endings
E. None of these Ref. 26 - p. 567

844. THE DORSAL COLUMN SYSTEM OF THE CENTRAL NERVOUS SYSTEM TRANSMITS SENSATIONS OF:
A. Pain
B. Temperature
C. Crude touch
D. Discriminative touch
E. Tickle and itch
Ref. 26 - p. 568

845. THE MOST IMPORTANT FUNCTIONAL CHARACTERISTIC OF THE DORSAL COLUMN PATHWAY IS THE:
A. Slowness of transmission
B. Transmission of accurate peripheral information
C. Diffusion of cortical impulses
D. Much alteration of impulses from other areas of the nervous system
E. Lack of proportionate relation between stimulus and cortical response
Ref. 26 - p. 571

846. WHEN IMPULSES ARE TRANSMITTED IN THE DORSAL COLUMN PATHWAY:
A. All the cortical neurons of a single receptor stimulus discharge at the same rate
B. Cortical neurons in the peripheral cortical "field" discharge most
C. Cortical neurons in the central part of the cortical "field" discharge most
D. A weak stimulus causes only peripheral neurons in the cortical "field" to fire
E. A strong stimulus causes only localized response in the cortex
Ref. 26 - p. 572

847. CHARACTERISTIC OF THE SPINOTHALAMIC SYSTEM IS ITS:
A. Rapid transmission of impulses
B. Highly discrete localization of sensory signals
C. Transmission of 2-point discrimination impulses
D. Transmission of crude touch and pressure sensations
E. Transmission of vibratory sensations
Ref. 26 - p. 573

848. CHARACTERISTIC OF DERMATOMES IS THEIR:
A. Innervation by one spinal nerve
B. Overlap of segmental fields of skin
C. Lack of significant loss of sensation with destruction of one spinal cord posterior root
D. All of the above
E. None of the above Ref. 26 - p. 575

849. INVESTIGATORS OF VARIATION IN PAIN TOLERANCE AMONG PEOPLE HAVE FOUND:
A. Some persons unusually sensitive to pain
B. Some persons unusually insensitive to pain
C. Eskimos, Indians and whites show significant differences in thresholds for pain
D. Eskimos, Indians and whites show no significant differences in thresholds for pain
E. A and C Ref. 26 - p. 578

850. STUDIES OF WOUNDED SOLDIERS HAVE SHOWN THAT:
A. Pain is generally felt while damage is being done
B. Pain is generally felt after damage has been done
C. Pain is generally not felt after damage has been done
D. Pain resulting from heat is not correlated with the ability of heat to damage tissue
E. Tissues are not destroyed if exposed indefinitely to temperature of 45° C. Ref. 26 - p. 578

851. ALL OF THE FOLLOWING ARE CHARACTERISTIC OF PAIN RECEPTORS, EXCEPT THAT THEY ARE:
A. Free nerve endings
B. Widespread in superficial layers of skin
C. Widespread in periosteum and joint surfaces
D. Encapsulated receptors
E. Widespread in arterial walls Ref. 26 - p. 578

852. POSTULATED MECHANISMS FOR ELICITING PAIN CONSIST OF ALL, EXCEPT:
A. Release of histamine by damaged cells
B. Tissue ischemia
C. Muscle spasm
D. Vasodilation
E. Release of proteolytic enzymes which split substances from globulin
Ref. 26 - p. 579

853. INVESTIGATORS OF THE SENSATION OF PAIN HAVE FOUND:
A. Removal of cortical sensory areas destroys pain perception
B. Pain impulses can be perceived at the level of the thalamus
C. No conscious perception of pain is possible lower in the CNS than the thalamus
D. Stimulation of somatic sensory area II does not elicit pain
E. Somatic area I is more concerned with pain sensation than somatic sensory area II
Ref. 26 - p. 581

854. ALL OF THE FOLLOWING ARE CHARACTERISTIC OF VISCERAL PAIN, EXCEPT:
A. Viscera have sensory receptors only for pain
B. Highly localized types of damage to viscera rarely cause severe pain
C. Diffuse stimulation of visceral pain nerve endings may cause severe pain
D. Ischemia of gut may cause extreme pain
E. Highly localized damage to the gut often causes severe pain
Ref. 26 - p. 582

855. THE THALAMIC SYNDROME USUALLY CONSISTS OF ALL THE FOLLOWING, EXCEPT:
A. Loss of almost all sensations from opposite side of body
B. Ataxia
C. Tic douloureux
D. Painful sensations resulting from strong stimuli
E. Perception of many affective unpleasant sensations
Ref. 26 - p. 586

856. WHICH OF THE FOLLOWING IS NOT CHARACTERISTIC OF THERMAL SENSATIONS?:
A. No specific complex receptors for either heat or cold
B. Great capacity for adaptation
C. Marked response to changes in surface temperature
D. Direct response to temperature of the receptor itself
E. Response to temperature gradients between different depths of skin
Ref. 26 - pp. 589-590

857. ALL THE FOLLOWING FACTS ARE TRUE ABOUT THE ATTENUATING REFLEX OF THE EAR, EXCEPT IT:
A. Occurs after a latent period of 10 milliseconds
B. Results from contraction of both stapedius and tensor tympani
C. Results from contraction of stapedius only
D. Reduces transmission of low frequency sound to the cochlea
E. Protects cochlea from damage by excessively loud noise
Ref. 26 - p. 593

858. FUNCTION OF THE BASILAR MEMBRANE OF THE COCHLEA HAS ALL THE FOLLOWING FEATURES, EXCEPT:
A. High frequency resonance occurring near the base
B. High frequency resonance occurring near the apex
C. Volume elasticity of the fibers near the helicotrema 100 times as great as at the base
D. A low frequency sound wave travels the entire distance along the membrane before it dies
E. A sound wave travels progressively slower as it moves into the cochlea Ref. 26 - p. 594

859. THE NERVOUS SYSTEM DETECTS DIFFERENT PITCHES BY:
A. The place principle
B. Differences in electrical potential
C. Activation of large numbers of neurons by various pitches
D. All of the above
E. None of the above Ref. 26 - p. 597

860. WHICH OF THE FOLLOWING ARE NOT INVOLVED IN DETERMINATION OF LOUDNESS BY THE AUDITORY SYSTEM?:
A. Amplitude of vibration of basilar membrane and hair cells
B. Rapidity of excitation of hair cells
C. Number of hair cells stimulated
D. Spatial summation of impulses
E. Place principle Ref. 26 - p. 598

861. IN THE AUDITORY AREAS OF THE CEREBRAL CORTEX, ALL BUT WHICH OF THE FOLLOWING IS TRUE?:
A. Short latency areas are directly excited by projections from the medial geniculate
B. Long latency areas are excited secondarily by impulses from short latency areas
C. Long latency areas are excited by projections from the medial geniculate
D. Short latency areas are secondary auditory cortex
E. Long latency areas are secondary auditory cortex
Ref. 26 - p. 600

862. BILATERAL DESTRUCTION OF THE AUDITORY CORTEX IN AN ANIMAL RESULTS IN:
A. Complete deafness
B. Reduction of discrimination of different patterns of sound
C. Possible abolishment of discrimination of tonal patterns
D. Inability to recognize previously learned sequence of tones
E. All of the above Ref. 26 - p. 601

863. WHEN SOUND ENTERS ONE EAR SLIGHTLY BEFORE IT ENTERS THE OTHER EAR:
A. It excites neurons in the contralateral superior olivary nucleus
B. It inhibits neurons in the ipsilateral superior olivary nucleus
C. Portions of the superior olivary nucleus have longer time lags of inhibition than do others
D. All of the above Ref. 26 - p. 601

864. IN CONDUCTION DEAFNESS:
A. The VIIIth nerve is destroyed
B. The middle ear mechanisms are impaired
C. The cochlea is destroyed
D. All of the above
E. A and C Ref. 26 - p. 602

865. THE LENS SYSTEM OF THE EYE INCLUDES WHICH OF THE FOLLOWING?:
A. Interface between air and anterior surface of the cornea
B. Interface between posterior surface of cornea and the aqueous humor
C. Interface between aqueous humor and anterior surface of lens
D. Interface between posterior surface of lens and vitreous humor
E. All of these Ref. 26 - p. 607

866. THE AREA OF GREATEST ACUITY OF VISUAL PERCEPTION IN THE RETINA IS THE:
A. Pigmented layer
B. Macula
C. Fovea
D. Ganglion layer
E. Peripheral cones
Ref. 26 - pp. 616, 626, 627

867. FUNCTION OF THE RODS OF THE RETINA RESULTS FROM:
A. Exposure to light
B. Decomposition of rhodopsin
C. Generation of a receptor potential
D. All of the above Ref. 26 - p. 618

868. NIGHT BLINDNESS IS ASSOCIATED WITH:
A. Vitamin A deficiency
B. Depression of quantities of retinene in the rods
C. Depression of quantities of rhodopsin in the rods
D. Depression of color photosensitive chemicals in the cones
E. All of the above Ref. 26 - p. 619

869. THE OPTIC PATHWAY CONSISTS OF ALL BUT THE FOLLOWING:
A. Optic nerve
B. Hypothalamus
C. Lateral geniculate body
D. Optic radiation
E. Visual cortex Ref. 26 - p. 626

870. ALL OF THE FOLLOWING STATEMENTS ARE TRUE REGARDING GANGLION CELLS OF THE RETINA, EXCEPT:
A. Transmit impulses at a rate of about 5/sec. even in total darkness
B. Transmit continuous nerve impulses
C. Respond to a spot of light with intense transient discharge
D. When light is turned off, the spot of cells responds with intense discharge
E. Concentric area of cells surrounding spot of light are an "inhibited area" Ref. 26 - p. 628

871. THE FUNCTION OF THE VISUAL CORTEX IS CONCERNED WITH:
A. Contrasts in the visual scene
B. Patterns of contrast
C. Detection of orientation of lines or borders
D. All of these Ref. 26 - p. 630

872. THE PRIMARY VISUAL CORTEX IS STRONGLY EXCITED BY ALL, EXCEPT:
A. Sudden changes in light intensity
B. Perception of steady signals
C. Changes in light intensity along borders
D. Movement of an image across the retina
E. A brief rapid discharge of ganglion cells following initial stimulation
Ref. 26 - p. 631

873. CONJUGATE MOVEMENTS OF THE EYES ARE THOUGHT TO BE CONTROLLED BY THE:
A. Parietal lobe
B. Superior colliculus
C. Temporal lobe
D. Pretectal region
E. Lateral geniculate
Ref. 26 - pp. 633-634

874. DETERMINATION OF INTACT PARASYMPATHETIC NERVES TO THE EYE CAN BE MADE BY THE FOLLOWING RESPONSE OF THE PUPIL TO LIGHT:
A. Convergence
B. Miosis
C. Mydriasis
D. Argyll Robertson pupil
E. All of the above
Ref. 26 - p. 637

875. ALL OF THE FOLLOWING ARE CHARACTERISTICS OF HORNER'S SYNDROME, EXCEPT:
A. Constricted pupil
B. Dilated pupil
C. Droop of superior eyelid
D. Persistent dilation of facial blood vessels
E. Lack of sweating on the affected side of face and head
Ref. 26 - p. 638

876. CHEMICALS CAUSING THE PRIMARY SENSATIONS OF TASTE ARE CORRECTLY RELATED IN THE FOLLOWING ITEMS, EXCEPT:
A. Sour taste by acids
B. Sweet taste by organic substances
C. Salty taste by ionized salts
D. Bitter taste by acids
E. Bitter taste by alkaloids
Ref. 26 - pp. 639-640

877. THE TASTE SENSE MOST SENSITIVE TO STIMULI IS:
A. Sour
B. Salty
C. Sweet
D. Bitter
Ref. 26 - p. 640

878. WHICH OF THE FOLLOWING IS CHARACTERISTIC OF ADAPTATION OF TASTE BUDS?:
A. Is rapid during the first 2-3 seconds of taste stimulus
B. First burst of impulses allows detection of minute concentrations of taste substances
C. Normal concentrations of taste substances cause prolonged discharge of taste fibers
D. Extreme adaptation is thought to occur in the central nervous system
E. All of these Ref. 26 - p. 642

879. THE NECESSARY STIMULI FOR SMELL MUST HAVE ALL THE FOLLOWING CHARACTERISTICS, EXCEPT:
A. Be volatile
B. Have threshold concentration
C. Be water soluble
D. Be lipid soluble
E. Be chemically acid Ref. 26 - p. 644

880. THE GAMMA EFFERENT FIBERS ASSOCIATED WITH THE MUSCLE SPINDLE:
A. Average 5 μ in diameter
B. Cause contraction of intrafusal muscle fibers
C. Reduce excitation of the muscle spindle
D. All of these
E. A and B Ref. 26 - p. 649

881. FIBERS FROM THE SECONDARY (FLOWER-SPRAY) RECEPTORS:
A. Terminate directly on the anterior motoneurons of the spinal cord
B. Have collaterals which synapse in the dorsal cord and send second order fibers up the spinocerebellar tracts
C. Cause delayed cerebellar reflexes
D. Terminate principally on internuncial cells of the spinal cord
E. Average approximately 15 μ in diameter
Ref. 26 - pp. 649-650

882. THE MYOTATIC OR STRETCH REFLEX:
A. Employs several neurons
B. Employs only two neurons
C. Is initiated by stretch of the primary receptor of the muscle spindle
D. All of these
E. All except A Ref. 26 - p. 650

883. THE DYNAMIC STRETCH REFLEX:
A. Is caused by continuous stretch
B. Follows sudden increase in stretch
C. Inhibits muscle tone
D. All of these Ref. 26 - p. 651

884. WHICH OF THE FOLLOWING ARE NOT TRUE IN RELATION TO MUSCLE SPINDLE ACTION?:
A. Contraction of the intrafusal fibers stretches the primary receptor
B. The receptor transmits excitatory impulses to the motoneuron
C. Action in B causes large muscle fibers to contract
D. The receptor sends continual impulses after the spindle returns to normal length
E. The skeletal muscle adjusts automatically to the length of the spindle
Ref. 26 - pp. 651-652

885. IF PRESSURE IS APPLIED TO THE SIDE, FRONT, OR BACK OF THE FOOT, THE FOOT MOVES IN THE DIRECTION OF THE PRESSURE APPLIED. THIS REACTION IS THE
A. Righting reflex
B. Mark time reflex
C. Positive supporting reaction
D. Magnet reaction
E. Rebound Ref. 26 - p. 658

886. THE BULBORETICULAR FACILITATORY AREA HAS ALL BUT ONE OF THE FOLLOWING CHARACTERISTICS:
A. Stimulation results in general increase in muscle tone
B. Located only in the medulla
C. If uninhibited, transmits continuous nerve impulses
D. Receives inhibitory signals from basal ganglia
E. Causes rigidity of skeletal muscles when higher portions of the nervous system are removed Ref. 26 - p. 663

887. WHICH OF THE FOLLOWING DOES NOT RESULT FROM STIMULATION OF THE SEMICIRCULAR CANALS?:
A. Detection of linear acceleration
B. Detection of angular acceleration
C. Nystagmus
D. All of these
E. None of these Ref. 26 - pp. 665, 666, 667

888. THE MOST IMPORTANT PROPRIOCEPTIVE INFORMATION NEEDED FOR THE MAINTENANCE OF EQUILIBRIUM IS DERIVED FROM THE:
A. Vestibular apparatus
B. Proprioceptors of the body
C. Exteroceptive sensations
D. Joint receptors of the neck
E. Visual mechanisms Ref. 26 - p. 668

889. THE SUBTHALAMIC AREA FUNCTIONS PARTICULARLY IN RELATION TO:
A. Inhibition of motor tone
B. Forward progression
C. Gross intentional movements
D. Equilibrium
E. Righting Ref. 26 - p. 670

890. DAMAGE TO THE BASAL GANGLIA MAY RESULT IN ANY OF THE FOLLOWING, EXCEPT:
A. Extraneous, involuntary movements
B. Rigidity
C. Tremor
D. Flaccid paralysis
E. Loss of automatic, associated movements
Ref. 26 - pp. 672-673

891. WHICH OF THE FOLLOWING FUNCTIONS DOES NOT REQUIRE AN INTACT CEREBRAL CORTEX?:
A. Visual righting reflex
B. Walking with normal progression
C. Purposefulness of locomotion
D. Hopping reaction
E. Placing reaction
Ref. 26 - p. 674

892. REPRESENTATION OF MUSCLES IN THE MOTOR PORTION OF THE CEREBRAL CORTEX IS GREATEST FOR THE:
A. Shoulder
B. Knee
C. Trunk
D. Face
E. Hand
Ref. 26 - p. 679

893. FUNCTIONS OF THE CEREBELLUM INCLUDE ALL THE FOLLOWING, EXCEPT:
A. Initiation of motor activities
B. Control of rate and timing of movement
C. Automatic excitation of antagonistic muscles at the end of a movement
D. "Damping" of muscular movements
E. Control of orderly sequence from one movement to another
Ref. 26 - pp. 684, 685, 686

894. THE FOLLOWING FIBERS ARE SAID TO BE CHOLINERGIC:
A. Preganglionic sympathetic neurons
B. Preganglionic parasympathetic neurons
C. Postganglionic parasympathetic neurons
D. All of these
E. None of these
Ref. 26 - p. 694

895. STIMULATION OF THE ADRENAL MEDULLA RESULTS IN:
A. Secretion of epinephrine and norepinephrine
B. Release of hormones with almost the same effects as direct sympathetic stimulation
C. Indirect stimulation of the sympathetics
D. All of these
E. None of these
Ref. 26 - pp. 697-698

896. WHICH OF THE FOLLOWING ARE SYMPATHETIC REFLEXES?:
A. Baroreceptor reflex
B. Gastrointestinal reflexes
C. Bladder emptying reflex
D. All of these
E. None of these
Ref. 26 - pp. 699-700

897. RESULTS OF STIMULATION OF VARIOUS PARTS OF THE HYPOTHALAMUS INCLUDE ALL OF THE FOLLOWING, EXCEPT:
A. Changes in arterial blood pressure
B. Changes in heart rate
C. Painful sensations
D. Extreme hunger or loss of desire for food
E. Initiation of rage reaction Ref. 26 - p. 703

898. THE RETICULAR ACTIVATING SYSTEM IS LOCATED IN THE:
A. Brain stem
B. Mesencephalon
C. Thalamus
D. Cerebral cortex
E. All of these
Ref. 26 - p. 705

899. IT IS BELIEVED THAT THE PORTION OF THE RETICULAR ACTIVATING SYSTEM BASICALLY RESPONSIBLE FOR NORMAL WAKEFULNESS IS THE:
A. Brain stem
B. Thalamus
C. Hypothalamus
D. Cerebral cortex Ref. 26 - p. 705

900. FUNCTION OF THE PRIMARY SOMATIC SENSORY AREA OF THE CEREBRAL CORTEX IS TO:
A. Receive visual impulses
B. Receive auditory impulses
C. Analyze motor activity
D. Analyze only simple aspects of somatic sensations
E. Analyze intricate patterns of sensory experience
Ref. 26 - p. 718

901. DESTRUCTION OF BOTH TEMPORAL LOBES RESULTS IN LOSS OF:
A. Interpretation of somatic sensations
B. Recent memory
C. Sight
D. Motor function
E. All of these Ref. 26 - p. 720

902. THE MOST IMPORTANT CORTICAL AREA OF THE DOMINANT HEMISPHERE FOR ORIGIN OF THE THOUGHT OF A MOTOR ACTIVITY IS THE:
A. Premotor area
B. Primary motor area
C. Superior temporal gyrus and angular gyrus
D. Occipital lobe
E. Prefrontal region Ref. 26 - p. 727

903. STIMULATION OF THE AMYGDALA CAUSES ALL OF THE FOLLOWING RESULTS, EXCEPT:
A. Same as those of hypothalamus
B. Tonic movements
C. Changes in respiration
D. Epileptic seizures
E. Sexual activities Ref. 26 - p. 733

904. ALL OF THE FOLLOWING ARE TRUE ABOUT THE KLUVER-BUCY SYNDROME, EXCEPT:
A. It results from removal of the anterior parietal cortex
B. Animal has excessive tendency to examine objects
C. Characterized by loss of fear
D. Animal shows decreased aggressiveness
E. Changes in dietary habits result Ref. 26 - p. 734

905. WHICH OF THE FOLLOWING IS NOT TRUE IN RELATION TO THE NERVE MEMBRANE POTENTIAL?:
A. All points on the surface of uninjured resting surface are isopotential
B. An injured part of the protoplasmic structure is electrically negative to the uninjured part
C. An injured part of the protoplasmic structure is electrically positive to the uninjured part
D. Intact nerve and muscle fibers exhibit a steady difference of electrical potential across their membranes
E. The exterior of the nerve fiber is positive in relation to the interior
Ref. 27 - p. 55

906. AN ACTION POTENTIAL IS CHARACTERIZED BY:
A. Depolarization of the resting membrane
B. Active region of the membrane surface is electrically positive
C. Inactive region of the membrane surface is electrically negative
D. A spike or overshoot
E. A and D Ref. 27 - pp. 58-59

907. PROPAGATION OF AN ACTION POTENTIAL ALONG THE NERVE FIBER IS:
A. A stimulus artifact
B. Different in various types of nerve fibers
C. Dependent on the original stimulus
D. The nerve impulse
E. None of these Ref. 27 - p. 59

908. ALL OF THE FOLLOWING ARE TRUE IN RELATION TO INTENSITY OF STIMULI, EXCEPT:
A. A threshold stimulus is subliminal
B. A liminal stimulus is a measure of the irritability of the tissue
C. At a particular value of stimulus strength, the amplitude of response becomes fixed
D. Up to maximal stimulus action potential amplitude increases
Ref. 27 - p. 61

909. WHEN A MAXIMAL STIMULUS IS APPLIED TO A NERVE TRUNK:
A. Only a portion of the nerve fibers are excited
B. Above threshold stimulus, action potential is dependent on stimulus strength
C. Individual fibers follow the law of all-or-none
D. Threshold stimulus produces a constant nerve impulse independent of environmental factors
E. All of these Ref. 27 - p. 61

910. BASIS FOR THE STRENGTH-DURATION CURVE IS THAT:
A. No relation exists between stimulus strength and excitation time
B. The stronger the stimulus, the shorter the excitation time
C. The weaker the stimulus, the shorter the excitation time
D. The rheobase is subliminal strength
E. None of these Ref. 27 - pp. 61-62

911. DURING A CONTINUED CONSTANT FLOW OF CURRENT ALONG A NERVE:
A. Additional impulses are generated
B. Fatigue occurs
C. Accommodation occurs
D. No additional impulses are generated
E. C and D Ref. 27 - p. 62

912. TEMPORAL SUMMATION IS:
A. Not related to strength of stimulus
B. Summation of subliminal stimuli
C. Summation of liminal stimuli
D. Decreases local excitatory state
E. None of these Ref. 27 - p. 63

913. IF A SECOND ADEQUATE STIMULUS IS SENT INTO A NERVE FOLLOWING GENERATION OF ONE ACTION POTENTIAL, THE EFFECTS INCLUDE ALL BUT:
A. An increase in excitability
B. A decrease in excitability
C. An absolute refractory period
D. A relatively refractory period
E. Recovery with temporary hyperexcitability
Ref. 27 - p. 63

914. WHEN A NERVE IS STIMULATED SOMEWHERE IN ITS COURSE:
A. The impulse can travel only in one direction
B. Dromic stimulation of a motor nerve causes the impulse to travel away from the muscle
C. Dromic stimulation of a motor nerve causes the impulse to travel toward the muscle
D. A and B
E. A and C Ref. 27 - p. 64

915. NERVE IMPULSE VELOCITY:
A. For a given fiber varies with stimulus strength
B. Is greatest in C type fibers
C. Usually varies directly with diameter of the fiber
D. In mammals is most rapid in non-medullated fibers
E. None of these Ref. 27 - pp. 66-67

916. A MYELIN SHEATH AROUND NERVE FIBERS:
A. Has no effect on propagation velocity
B. Has pronounced effect on propagation velocity
C. Is interrupted by nodes of Ranvier
D. C only
E. B and C Ref. 27 - p. 67

917. ALL OF THE FOLLOWING ARE TRUE ABOUT SALTATORY CONDUCTION, EXCEPT:
A. Local current flow is restricted to region of nodes of Ranvier
B. Occurs in myelinated nerves
C. Is a continuous wavelike impulse propagation
D. Provides for rapid conduction velocity
E. Depolarization of only a fraction of the axon membrane during activity
Ref. 27 - p. 67

918. MAGNITUDE OF ACTION POTENTIAL AND VELOCITY OF THE IMPULSE ARE BOTH DECREASED BY ALL OF THE FOLLOWING, EXCEPT:
A. Ether
B. Cold
C. Fatigue
D. Hypoxia
E. Atmosphere of nitrogen
Ref. 27 - p. 69

919. PROPAGATION OF AN IMPULSE BY A NERVE DIFFERS FROM THAT OF CONDUCTION OF AN ELECTRICAL CURRENT BY A WIRE IN ALL THE FOLLOWING WAYS, EXCEPT THAT THE NERVE FIBER:
A. Is an active agent
B. Energy comes from the nerve itself
C. Impulse strength is maintained at a constant level
D. Impulse velocity is greater
E. Has none of the above
Ref. 27 - pp. 69-70

920. INVESTIGATION HAS FOUND THAT ELECTRICAL SYNAPSES:
A. Occur in mammalian nervous systems
B. Have similar structure to chemical synapses
C. Have cell membranes in close proximity
D. Show high intercellular resistance
E. Utilize acetylcholine transmitter
Ref. 27 - p. 70

921. CHEMICAL SYNAPSES SHOW ALL THE FOLLOWING CHARACTERISTICS, EXCEPT:
A. Release of a transmitter
B. A narrow cleft between presynaptic and postsynaptic membranes
C. Numerous mitochondria of presynaptic cell
D. Many synaptic vesicles
E. A decrease in permeability of the postsynaptic cell membrane
Ref. 27 - p. 70

922. WHICH OF THE FOLLOWING STATEMENTS ARE TRUE ABOUT THE AUTONOMIC NERVOUS SYSTEM?:
A. Pathways consist of two neurons
B. Neuronal fibers traverse anterior roots of spinal cord
C. Preganglionic fibers synapse in an autonomic ganglion
D. Collateral ganglion may receive preganglionic fibers
E. All of these
Ref. 27 - p. 202

923. MUSCLE INNERVATED BY THE AUTONOMIC NERVES:
A. Consists of skeletal muscle
B. Neuromuscular transmission is cholinergic
C. All muscle cells are innervated
D. Noninnervated cells may be excited by electrotonic coupling
E. None of these
Ref. 27 - p. 202

924. THE SYMPATHETIC NERVOUS SYSTEM HAS ITS SOURCE IN THE:
A. Thoracolumbar spinal cord
B. Midbrain
C. Medulla oblongata
D. Sacral cord segments
E. Cervical cord segments Ref. 27 - p. 203

925. SPLANCHNIC NERVES ARE:
A. Composed of parasympathetic fibers
B. Composed of postganglionic sympathetic fibers
C. Composed of preganglionic sympathetics
D. Always synapse in paravertebral ganglia
E. Only C and D Ref. 27 - p. 203

926. PARASYMPATHETIC NEURONS:
A. Have long postganglionic fibers
B. Have short postganglionic fibers
C. Have ganglia distant to the organ innervated
D. Form the thoracic splanchnic nerves
E. Innervate muscle in the limbs Ref. 27 - p. 203

927. THE INTEGRATIVE CENTER FOR THE VISCERAL FUNCTIONS GOVERNED BY THE AUTONOMIC NERVOUS SYSTEM IS THE:
A. Cerebral cortex
B. Spinal cord
C. Midbrain
D. Hypothalamus
E. Thalamus
Ref. 27 - p. 207

928. ALL OF THE FOLLOWING ARE CHOLINERGIC NERVES, EXCEPT:
A. Preganglionic sympathetics
B. Preganglionic parasympathetics
C. Postganglionic sympathetics
D. Postganglionic parasympathetics
E. Nerves to sweat glands Ref. 27 - p. 207

THE FOLLOWING ARE SYMPTOMS FOLLOWING STIMULATION OF A NERVE TO THE HEART:

1. Cardiac inhibition
2. Release of acetylcholine
3. Fall in blood pressure
4. Fainting

929. WHICH OF THE FOLLOWING NERVES HAS BEEN STIMULATED?:
A. Phrenic
B. Sympathetic nerves
C. Vagus
D. Splanchnic nerve Ref. 27 - p. 266

930. THE CARDIAC INHIBITORY CENTER IS LOCATED IN THE:
A. Spinal cord
B. Medulla
C. Midbrain
D. Thalamus
E. Cerebral cortex
Ref. 27 - p. 266

931. IN THE CAROTID SINUS REFLEX:
A. Afferent impulses travel via the glossopharyngeal nerve
B. The heart is slowed
C. The stimulus is increased blood pressure
D. The carotid sinus nerve endings are pressoreceptors
E. All of these are true Ref. 27 - p. 268

932. SECTIONING OF BOTH VAGUS NERVES RESULTS IN:
A. Cardiac acceleration
B. Cardiac deceleration
C. Presence of the aortic reflex
D. Stimulation of the cardioinhibitory center
E. Fall in blood pressure Ref. 27 - p. 269

933. NERVES CONSTRICTING SMOOTH MUSCLE IN THE BLOOD VESSELS ARE:
A. Parasympathetic vasoconstrictors
B. Parasympathetic vasodilators
C. Preganglionic sympathetics
D. Postganglionic sympathetics
E. Only A and C Ref. 27 - p. 272

934. ALL OF THE FOLLOWING CHARACTERIZE VASOMOTOR TONE, EXCEPT:
A. Large influence on blood pressure
B. Modification by sensory impulses from the body surfaces
C. Influenced by higher brain centers
D. Chemical stimulation by blood compounds
E. Independence of the vasomotor center
Ref. 27 - pp. 275-276

935. SUBSTANCES WHICH CAUSE DILATION OF BLOOD VESSELS BY INFLUENCING THE VASOMOTOR MECHANISM ARE:
A. Carbon dioxide
B. Epinephrine
C. Histamine
D. A and B
E. B and C
Ref. 27 - pp. 279-280

936. INNERVATION OF THE LARGE INTESTINE IS PROVIDED BY ALL THE FOLLOWING, EXCEPT:
A. Vagal supply to proximal colon
B. Sympathetic supply for stimulation of activity
C. Parasympathetic supply from sacral cord
D. Sympathetic supply for inhibition of activity
E. Parasympathetic supply for stimulation of activity
Ref. 27 - p. 366

937. INNERVATION OF SWEAT GLANDS IS:
A. By the sympathetic nervous system
B. By the parasympathetic nervous system
C. Influenced by a sweat center in the brain
D. All of these
E. Only A and C Ref. 27 - pp. 439-440

938. A HEAT REGULATING CENTER:
A. Is located in the thalamus
B. Is located in the hypothalamus
C. Is influenced by temperature of the circulating blood
D. Is influenced reflexly from the skin
E. B, C and D Ref. 27 - pp. 445-446

939. EFFECTS OF INJECTED EPINEPHRINE ON THE BODY INCLUDE ALL BUT:
A. Awareness to the environment is increased
B. Reflex responses are facilitated
C. Inhibitory effect on the central nervous system
D. Increase in heart rate
E. Effect on smooth muscle Ref. 27 - pp. 458-459

940. ALL OF THE FOLLOWING ARE TRUE ABOUT RECEPTORS, EXCEPT:
A. They are transducers
B. Each produces a depolarization of its membrane
C. Each produces a generator or receptor potential
D. Receptor potentials are propagated
E. Receptor membranes show nonselective permeability to all small ions
Ref. 27 - p. 110

941. FACTS RELATING TO ADAPTATION OF SENSORY RECEPTORS INCLUDE ALL, EXCEPT:
A. Receptor potential declines upon maintained stimulation
B. Adaptation is the result of fatigue
C. Phasic receptors are quickly adapting
D. Tonic receptors are slowly adapting
E. An "off" response is commonly a brief hyperpolarization
Ref. 27 - p. 110

942. THE FREQUENCY OF ACTION POTENTIALS FOLLOWING STIMULATION OF A RECEPTOR IS:
A. Commonly a function of the generator potential amplitude
B. Increased by adaptation
C. Proportional to the logarithm of the stimulus intensity
D. B and C
E. A and C Ref. 27 - pp. 110-111

943. THE LAW OF SPECIFIC NERVE ENERGIES STATES THAT:
A. Nature of modality is determined by the manner of stimulation
B. The modality of a sensation aroused by stimulation of a given sense organ is fixed
C. Coding of information contained in the specific stimulus always occurs
D. Different receptors for the same sensation have varied thresholds
Ref. 27 - p. 111

944. WEBER'S LAW STATES THAT:
A. The nature of modality is not determined by the manner in which the sense organ is stimulated
B. In the central nervous system an impulse can pass only in one direction
C. The least perceptible increase in the intensity of a stimulus is a constant fraction of the original stimulus
D. Sensations are invariably projected to the brain
Ref. 27 - p. 112

945. RECEPTIVE FIELDS FOR THE CUTANEOUS SENSATIONS:
A. Have size varying with the part of the body
B. Show the phenomenon of divergence
C. Show the phenomenon of convergence
D. All of these
E. None of these Ref. 27 - pp. 113-114

946. THE FOLLOWING OBSERVATIONS MAKE IT LIKELY THAT DISTINCT NERVES MEDIATE THE VARIOUS CUTANEOUS SENSATIONS, EXCEPT:
A. Punctiform manner of distribution in the skin
B. Application of cocaine to a cutaneous nerve causes touch to disappear first
C. Dissociation of cutaneous sensations in some pathological disturbances
D. Pressure on a nerve trunk may cause dissociation
E. Nerves with the smallest diameter are first affected by cocaine
Ref. 27 - p. 114

947. VISCERAL SENSATIONS IN THE INTERNAL ORGANS SHOW THAT THESE ORGANS:
A. Evidence no sense of touch, heat or cold
B. Are extremely sensitive to touch
C. Are extremely sensitive to heat
D. Are extremely sensitive to motion
E. B, C and D Ref. 27 - p. 118

948. THE FUNCTIONAL UNIT OF THE NERVOUS SYSTEM IS THE:
A. Neuron
B. Final common pathway
C. Brain and spinal cord
D. Spinal nerve
E. Reflex arc Ref. 27 - p. 123

949. ALL OF THE FOLLOWING STATEMENTS ARE TRUE ABOUT THE SYNAPSE, EXCEPT:
A. Neural contiguity but not continuity
B. Large numbers of mitochondria present in the presynaptic terminal
C. Degeneration of afferent neurons can extend across the synapse to the efferent neurons
D. Transmission of impulses in only one direction
E. Occurrence of a synaptic delay in passage of an impulse
Ref. 27 - pp. 124-125

950. EXCITATORY POSTSYNAPTIC POTENTIALS SHOW THE FOLLOWING CHARACTERISTIC:
A. A propagated action potential
B. A level of depolarization at about 10 mv. decline from resting potential
C. Excitation by temporal summation in the presynaptic fiber
D. Excitation by spatial summation in the presynaptic fiber
E. All of the above Ref. 27 - p. 125

951. INHIBITION AT THE SYNAPSE IS ACHIEVED BY:
A. Presynaptic but not postsynaptic inhibition
B. Postsynaptic but not presynaptic inhibition
C. Both presynaptic and postsynaptic inhibition
D. Transmitters which alter the membrane permeability to Na ions
E. Presynaptic inhibition of short duration
Ref. 27 - pp. 125-126

952. TRANSMITTERS IN THE CENTRAL NERVOUS SYSTEM INCLUDE:
A. Acetylcholine
B. Norepinephrine
C. Serotonin
D. Histamine
E. All of these
Ref. 27 - p. 126

953. CHARACTERISTICS OF REFLEXES INCLUDE ALL BUT:
A. In a spinal animal consistent stimuli produce consistent reflexes
B. In a normal animal consistent stimuli produce inconsistent reflexes
C. Reflex action is purposive
D. Reflex action is not adaptive
E. Reflex action is always of stereotyped nature
Ref. 27 - p. 127

954. IN EXPERIMENTAL REFLEX TIME OF A CAT, WHICH OF THE FOLLOWING CAN BE CALLED NUCLEAR DELAY?:
A. Total reflex time of 10.4 msec.
B. Conduction time over afferent and efferent nerves of 6.5 msec.
C. Time for passage through spinal cord polysynaptic pathways 3.9 msec.
D. B and C
E. Only A
Ref. 27 - p. 127

955. IN A CASE WHERE STIMULATION OF NERVE A BRINGS DISCHARGE OF 100 NEURONS IN A GIVEN POOL, AND STIMULATION OF NERVE B EXCITES 100 NEURONS, 50 OF WHICH WERE THE SAME AS THOSE RESPONDING SIMULTANEOUSLY IN NERVE A, THE RESPONSE INVOLVES ONLY 150 NEURONS. THIS IS AN EXAMPLE OF:
A. Central facilitation
B. Spatial summation
C. Integration
D. Occlusion
E. Central depression
Ref. 27 - p. 128

956. THE FINAL COMMON PATHWAY IS THE:
A. Afferent nerve
B. Efferent nerve
C. The reflex arc
D. The internuncial neurons
E. The muscle cell
Ref. 27 - p. 128

957. ALL OF THE FOLLOWING FACTS APPLY TO INHIBITION OF MUSCLE, EXCEPT:
A. Cardiac muscle is supplied with direct efferent inhibitory nerves
B. Skeletal muscle of vertebrates is supplied with inhibitory nerves
C. Intestinal muscle is supplied with direct inhibitory efferent nerves
D. Skeletal muscle of vertebrates has no inhibitory nerves
E. B and C
Ref. 27 - p. 130

958. THE MYOTATIC REFLEX CAN BE DISTINGUISHED FROM ALL OTHER REFLEXES BY THE FACT THAT:
A. It is stimulated by stretch receptors
B. It acts through the final common pathway
C. It is inhibitory to extensors
D. Its proprioceptive impulses return to the muscle in which they originated
E. Afterdischarge is present Ref. 27 - p. 134

959. STRETCH ON THE NUCLEAR BAG REGION OF THE MUSCLE SPINDLE RESULTS IN WHICH OF THE FOLLOWING?:
A. A regular discharge of impulses in the primary afferent
B. Contraction of extrafusal fibers through activation of alpha motoneurons
C. Reduction of spindle tension through contraction of extrafusal fibers
D. Rhythmic firing of stretch receptor
E. All of these Ref. 27 - pp. 136-137

960. RENSHAW CELLS ACT TO ACHIEVE:
A. Hypertonia
B. Excitation of motoneurons
C. Recurrent inhibition
D. Hypotonia
E. Myotatic reflex Ref. 27 - p. 138

961. THE IMPORTANCE OF THE GAMMA SYSTEM LIES IN ITS ABILITY TO:
A. Regulate the sensitivity of the spindle
B. Regulate the muscle total tension
C. Cause the polar regions of the spindle to lengthen
D. Decrease the firing rate of the spindle receptor
E. All of these Ref. 27 - p. 137

962. THE FOLLOWING FACTORS INFLUENCE THE TYPE AND FREQUENCY OF BRAIN WAVES:
A. Age
B. Area of the brain studied
C. Sleep
D. Types of brain pathology
E. All of these Ref. 27 - pp. 191-192

963. A PERSON WITH AN EMMETROPIC EYE HAS A CONDITION IN WHICH:
A. The posterior principal focus lies upon the retina when the eye is at rest
B. An object nearer than 20 ft. can be seen distinctly
C. He can see far objects by accommodation
D. All of these
E. None of these Ref. 27 - p. 146

964. WHEN THE EYE IS ACCOMMODATED:
A. The lens has less refractive power
B. Suspensory ligaments are relaxed
C. The lens assumes a more spherical form
D. The nearest point of focus is the near point of vision
E. B, C and D Ref. 27 - pp. 147-148

965. THE OPTIC DISC OF THE RETINA IS:
A. A blind spot
B. The fovea
C. The yellow spot
D. None of these
E. B and C
Ref. 27 - p. 154

966. ALL OF THE FOLLOWING PROCESSES TAKE PLACE IN THE RETINAL CELLS, EXCEPT:
A. Convergence
B. Divergence
C. Scotopic vision at the fovea
D. Intraretinal association
E. Facilitation
F. Inhibition
Ref. 27 - pp. 155-157

967. IN A SCOTOPIC EYE ALL THE FOLLOWING ARE TRUE, EXCEPT:
A. The fovea is blind
B. Colors are readily discernible
C. The eye is color blind
D. Red objects are not seen at all
E. Vision is twilight vision
Ref. 27 - p. 156

968. ACUTE HEARING DEPENDS ON:
A. Proper transmission of sound waves
B. Generation of nerve impulses in the organ of Corti
C. Transmission of impulses to the cerebral occipital lobe
D. All of these
E. Only A and B
Ref. 27 - pp. 169-189

969. THE AUDITORY NERVE:
A. Contains some efferent fibers
B. Contains no efferent fibers
C. Motor activity increases afferent action potentials
D. Only B
E. A and C
Ref. 27 - p. 170

970. ALL THE FOLLOWING STATEMENTS ABOUT CONDITIONED REFLEXES (CR) ARE TRUE, EXCEPT:
A. Conditioned stimulus can follow the unconditioned stimulus (US)
B. Are never acquired spontaneously
C. May occur simultaneously with the UR
D. Are always associated with an uncontitioned stimulus (US)
E. The shorter the lapse between US and conditioned stimulus, the quicker the CR is established
Ref. 27 - p. 196

971. WHICH OF THE FOLLOWING STATEMENTS IS TRUE ABOUT CONDITIONED REFLEXES?:
A. Summation is possible
B. Are susceptible to inhibition
C. Are inherited
D. Cerebral cortex is not essential
E. A and B
Ref. 27 - pp. 197-198

972. THE EYE IS SENSITIVE TO A BAND OF WAVELENGTHS OF THE SPECTRUM WHICH:
A. Are unequally effective in stimulating the retina
B. Are 723 mu to 397 mu
C. Determine hue or chroma
D. Influence intensity of light necessary to elicit a sensation
E. All of these Ref. 17 - p. 416

973. THE TYPES OF CHANGES IN ELECTRICAL POTENTIAL RECORDED FROM THE RETINA INCLUDE ALL BUT:
A. Steady corneoretinal potential
B. Phasic potential produced by light
C. Scotopic dominator response of cones
D. Unit responses from the level of the bipolar cells
E. Action potentials of ganglion cells and optic nerve fibers
Ref. 17 - pp. 420-421

974. SECTIONING OF THE OPTIC CHIASMA RESULTS IN:
A. Complete blindness of both eyes
B. Bitemporal hemianopsia
C. Unilateral nasal hemianopsia
D. Right homonymous hemianopsia
E. Left homonymous hemianopsia Ref. 17 - p. 444

975. WHEN LOCAL CURRENT FLOW IS ELICITED BY CHEMICAL OR MECHANICAL DEFORMATION OF NERVE ENDINGS, THE RESULTING ELECTRICAL VOLTAGES ARE CALLED:
A. Generator potentials
B. Receptor potentials
C. Action potentials
D. Specific nerve energies
E. Electromagnetic potentials Ref. 26 - p. 559

976. SIGNIFICANT FEATURES OF THE FUNCTION OF AUDITORY PATHWAYS ARE:
A. Rate of firing of single nerve fibers of Nerve VIII
B. Consistently synchronized firing of auditory tracts of brain with sound frequency
C. Transmission of unchanged sound signals from ear to brain
D. Continuance of low rates of impulse firing even in the absence of sound
E. All of these Ref. 26 - p. 599

977. TO DISCRIMINATE THE DIRECTION FROM WHICH SOUND COMES, THE TIME LAG BETWEEN ITS ENTRANCE INTO THE FIRST AND SECOND EAR IS:
A. The most discriminating factor for all frequencies
B. Functions best for freuqencies below 3000 cycles per second
C. Functions best for frequencies above 3000 cycles per second
D. More discriminating than intensity
E. Less discriminating than intensity Ref. 26 - p. 601

978. IN ACCOMMODATION OF THE EYE:
A. The ciliary muscle contracts
B. The ciliary muscle relaxes
C. Tension on the lens is released
D. Tension on the lens is increased
E. The lens assumes a more spherical shape
Ref. 26 - pp. 608-609

979. THE CILIARY MUSCLE OF THE EYE IS:
A. Controlled by the sympathetics
B. Controlled by the parasympathetics
C. Responsible for increasing refractive power of the lens
D. Controlled by the optic nerve
E. Responsible for accommodation for distant vision
Ref. 26 - p. 609

980. PRESBYOPIA IS A CONDITION OF THE EYES WHICH IS:
A. Frequently present in older individuals
B. Frequently present in young children
C. Near-sightedness
D. Far-sightedness
E. Decreased ability of the lens to accommodate
Ref. 26 - p. 609

981. THE LATERAL GENICULATE BODY HAS POSTULATED FUNCTIONS OF:
A. Relay of visual information to the visual cortex
B. A major role in fusion of vision
C. A part of the mechanism for stereoscopic visual depth perception
D. Accommodation
E. Pupillary light reflex
Ref. 26 - p. 629

982. THE PRIMARY VISUAL CORTICAL AREA LIES MAINLY IN THE:
A. Frontal lobe
B. Parietal lobe
C. Occipital lobe
D. Calcarine fissure
E. Angular gyrus
Ref. 26 - p. 629

983. FIXATION OF THE EYES ON SUCCESSIVE POINTS IN A CONTINUOUSLY MOVING SCENE IS:
A. Nystagmus
B. Fusion
C. Squint
D. Strabismus
E. Pursuit movement
Ref. 26 - pp. 634-635

984. RECEPTORS FOR TASTE SENSATION ARE TASTE BUDS WHICH:
A. Degenerate when taste nerve fibers are destroyed
B. Are not affected by age of the individual
C. Respond to a particular type of taste stimulus
D. Contain taste cells which stimulate taste nerve fibers
Ref. 26 - pp. 641-642

985. IN THE ANIMAL DECEREBRATED AT A LEVEL MIDWAY BETWEEN THE SUPERIOR AND INFERIOR COLLICULI:
A. Inhibitory influences from above are removed
B. The bulboreticular facilitatory area is removed
C. A high degree of facilitation is maintained in the cord
D. The animal has flaccid paralysis
E. All of these Ref. 26 - p. 647

986. IN A MOTOR UNIT:
A. A single nerve fiber is 9-16 μ in diameter
B. Most nerve fibers stimulate 100-300 skeletal muscle fibers
C. A motor neuron cell body is located in the posterior horn of the spinal cord
D. All of these
E. None of these Ref. 26 - p. 647

987. THE PRIMARY OR ANNULOSPINAL RECEPTORS OF THE MUSCLE SPINDLE:
A. Average 17 μ in diameter
B. Pass into the anterior roots of the spinal cord
C. Are highly sensitive to slight stretch
D. Depict rate of change of receptor length
E. Depict only the static length of the receptor itself
Ref. 26 - p. 649

988. THE GOLGI TENDON ORGAN:
A. Detects muscle length
B. Stimulates the individual muscle to contract
C. Detects muscle tension
D. Inhibits anterior motoneurons
E. All of these Ref. 26 - p. 650

989. WHICH OF THE FOLLOWING DOES NOT CHARACTERIZE THE GOLGI TENDON ORGAN REFLEX?:
A. Is excitatory
B. Is inhibitory
C. Involves inhibitory internuncial cells
D. Causes contraction of the entire muscle
E. Results in the "lengthening reaction"
Ref. 26 - p. 654

990. WHICH OF THE FOLLOWING ARE AUTONOMIC SEGMENTAL REFLEXES WHICH OCCUR IN THE SPINAL CORD?:
A. Vascular responses to heat and cold
B. Sweating
C. Pupillary light reflex
D. Dynamic stretch reflex
E. Emptying reflexes of the bladder Ref. 26 - p. 660

991. WHICH OF THE FOLLOWING DESCRIBE THE FLEXION REFLEX?:
A. Monosynaptic
B. Nociceptive
C. Diverging circuits
D. Repetitive after-discharge
E. Only two neurons Ref. 26 - pp. 650-651

992. SPECIFIC FUNCTIONS OF THE PREMOTOR AREA OF THE CEREBRAL CORTEX ARE THOUGHT TO BE:
A. Production of fine movement
B. Coordination of skilled movement
C. Discrete movements of the fingers
D. Acquisition of specialized motor skills
E. Eye movements for fixation of gaze Ref. 26 - p. 680

993. EFFECTS OF UNILATERAL TRANSECTION OF THE CORTICOSPINAL FIBERS AT THE LEVEL OF THE PYRAMIDS INCLUDE ALL BUT:
A. Loss of all discrete movements on the opposite side of the body
B. Hypotonia
C. Gradual atrophy of distal limb muscles
D. Loss of movements required for equilibrium
E. Loss of postural and fixation movements
Ref. 26 - pp. 681-682

994. INJURY OR REMOVAL OF PORTIONS OF THE CEREBELLUM WILL RESULT IN WHICH OF THE FOLLOWING?:
A. Intention tremor
B. Spasticity
C. Dysmetria
D. Loss of equilibrium
E. Hemiplegia
F. Hypotonia
G. Clonus
H. Past pointing Ref. 26 - p. 688

995. WHICH OF THE FOLLOWING CHARACTERIZE BRAIN WAVES?:
A. Intensities ranging from 0-300 microvolts
B. Character dependent on the degree of activity of the cerebral cortex
C. Generally regular patterns
D. Marked changes between states of sleep and wakefulness
E. Alpha waves which occur at frequencies of more than 14 cycles per second Ref. 26 - p. 711

996. THE MEANS BY WHICH THE VISUAL APPARATUS NORMALLY PERCEIVES DISTANCE ARE:
A. Relative sizes of objects
B. Spherical aberration
C. Moving parallax
D. Nystagmus
E. Stereopsis Ref. 26 - p. 613

997. WHICH OF THE FOLLOWING CHARACTERIZE HUMAN VISUAL ACTIVITY?:
A. Maximal acuity for discriminating between point sources of light is 26 seconds
B. Is greatest in the foveal region of the retina
C. Becomes greater as the periphery of the retina is reached
D. Two points of light with centers 0.5 micron apart on the retina can be distinguished
E. Becomes poorer as the periphery of the retina is reached
Ref. 26 - pp. 612-613

998. WHICH OF THE FOLLOWING STATEMENTS ARE TRUE ABOUT FUSION OF FLICKERING LIGHTS BY THE RETINA?:
A. The brighter the light, the lower the critical frequency for fusion
B. A flash of light excites visual receptors for 1/10 to 1/5 second
C. Persistence of excitation following stimulus
D. At a low intensity, critical frequency for fusion is 60 flashes per second
E. Successive flashes of light become fused
Ref. 26 - pp. 621-622

999. THE YOUNG-HELMHOLTZ THEORY EXPLAINS THAT:
A. Each of three types of rods respond maximally to a different color
B. Red, green and blue are the colors involved
C. Each of three types of cones respond maximally to a different color
D. Equal stimulation of all red, green and blue cones gives a sensation of seeing yellow
E. All of these
Ref. 26 - p. 622

FOR EACH OF THE FOLLOWING MULTIPLE CHOICE QUESTIONS, SELECT THE MOST APPROPRIATE ANSWER(S):

1000. WHERE ARE ENZYMES INVOLVED IN MONOAMINE BIOSYNTHESIS LOCALIZED?:
A. Neuron nucleus
B. Nucleolus
C. Golgi apparatus
D. Synaptosomes
E. Mitochondria
Ref. 19 - p. 48

1001. IT IS CURRENTLY BELIEVED THAT__________IS THE TRANSMITTER SUBSTANCE IN PERIPHERAL SYMPATHETIC NERVES:
A. Dopa
B. Epinephrine
C. Dopamine
D. Norepinephrine
E. Serotonin
Ref. 19 - p. 53

1002. __________IS THE PRECURSOR OF NOREPINEPHRINE AND IS ALSO A FINAL NEUROEFFECTOR IN THE NIGRO-NEOSTRIATE PATHWAY:
A. Dopamine
B. Tryptophan
C. Serotonin
D. Epinephrine
E. Histidine
Ref. 19 - p. 53

1003. THE CYTOPLASMIC PARTICLES OF THE ADRENAL MEDULLA ARE PRINCIPAL REPOSITORIES FOR:
A. Norepinephrine
B. Serotonin
C. Epinephrine
D. Dopamine
E. Dopa
Ref. 19 - p. 53

1004. WHAT IS THE RATE-LIMITING ENZYME IN THE FORMATION OF CATECHOLAMINES?:
A. Monoamine oxidase
B. Catechol-O-methyltransferase
C. Tyrosine hydroxylase
D. 3, 4-dihydroxyphenylalanine de carboxylase
E. Pyridoxal phosphate
Ref. 19 - p. 54

1005. CATECHOLAMINES ARE METABOLIZED PRIMARILY BY TWO OF THE FOLLOWING ENZYMES:
A. Dopamine-β-hydroxylase
B. Dopa decarboxylase
C. Monoamine oxidase
D. Catechol-O-methyltransferase
E. S-adenosylmethionine
Ref. 19 - p. 55

1006. MONOAMINE OXIDASE:
A. Is a mixture of different enzyme proteins
B. Is found complexed in the outer membrane of the mitochondrion
C. Requires enzyme-bound copper as a requisite for enzyme activity
D. Shows no substrate selectivity
E. May be provisionally separated into two groups by their sensitivity to carbonyl reagents
Ref. 19 - p. 55

1007. THE BIOSYNTHESIS OF 5-HT FROM L-TRYPTOPHAN PROCEEDS THROUGH WHICH OF THE FOLLOWING REACTIONS?:
A. Hydroxylation and decarboxylation
B. Hydroxylation alone
C. O-methylation
D. N-methylation
E. Decarboxylation alone
Ref. 19 - p. 67

1008. TEGMENTAL LESIONS IN MONKEYS AND RATS PRODUCED A DECREASE IN__________IN THE STRIATUM:
A. Serotonin
B. Dopamine
C. Epinephrine
D. Norepinephrine
E. 5-HT
Ref. 19 - p. 93

1009. LESIONS IN THE RAPHE NUCLEI OF CATS ARE FOLLOWED BY A DISAPPEARANCE OF BRAIN__________:
A. Serotonin
B. Dopamine
C. Epinephrine
D. Norepinephrine
E. 5-HT
Ref. 19 - p. 93

1010. LESIONS IN THE MIDDLE FOREBRAIN BUNDLE OF THE LATERAL HYPOTHALAMUS AND IN THE DORSOMEDIAL BRAIN STEM TEGMENTUM WILL SIGNIFICANTLY DECREASE BOTH__________ AND__________IN THE WHOLE RAT BRAIN:
A. Serotonin
B. Dopamine
C. Epinephrine
D. Norepinephrine
E. Dopa
Ref. 19 - p. 93

1011. SECTIONING THE THORACIC CORD IN A RAT WILL LEAD TO A DECREASE IN__________AND__________IN THE SPINAL CORD:
A. Serotonin
B. Dopamine
C. Epinephrine
D. Norepinephrine
E. Dopa
Ref. 19 - p. 93

1012. THE MAMMALIAN PINEAL CONTAINS RELATIVELY LARGE AMOUNTS OF WHICH OF THE FOLLOWING AMINES?:
A. Serotonin
B. Dopamine
C. Epinephrine
D. Norepinephrine
E. Dopa
Ref. 19 - p. 451

1013. THE SYNTHESIS, STORAGE, RELEASE AND METABOLISM OF CERTAIN COMPOUNDS IN PINEAL GLANDULAR CELLS APPEAR TO BE UNDER THE DIRECT CONTROL OF WHICH OF THE FOLLOWING NERVES?:
A. Vagus
B. Sympathetics
C. Glossopharyngeal
D. Parasympathetics
E. Facial
Ref. 19 - p. 451

1014. THE MAMMALIAN PINEAL IS OF SPECIAL INTEREST TO THE NEUROCHEMIST FOR WHICH OF THE FOLLOWING REASONS?:
A. High concentration of parasympathetic nerve endings
B. Contains no enzymes
C. Metabolic transformations which occur only within the pineal
D. Pineal serotonin varies as a function of time and light
E. Is easily separated from the rest of the brain
Ref. 19 - p. 451

1015. RECENT STUDIES OF THE UPTAKE OF TRITIATED ESTRADIOL, PROGESTERONE AND TESTOSTERONE IN THE BRAIN INDICATE THAT THE__________CONCENTRATES MORE LABELED STEROID:

A. Hippocampus
B. Cortex
C. Thalamus
D. Pineal
E. Hypothalamus

Ref. 19 - p. 436

1016. THE MOST IMPORTANT NEUROSECRETORY SYSTEMS IN VERTEBRATES ARE FOUND IN THE__________:

A. Pineal
B. Medulla
C. Septum
D. Amygdala
E. Hypothalamus

Ref. 19 - p. 378

1017. MORE THAN__________% OF THE SEROTONIN FORMED IN THE BRAIN IS EVENTUALLY ELIMINATED FROM BRAIN AS 5-HYDROXYINDOLEACETIC ACID (5-HIAA):

A. 20
B. 58
C. 70
D. 90
E. 40

Ref. 19 - p. 68

1018. WHICH OF THE FOLLOWING AMINO ACIDS PROBABLY ACT AS STRONG INHIBITORY TRANSMITTERS?:

A. L-glutamate
B. Glycine
C. GABA
D. L-aspartate
E. Serine

Ref. 19 - p. 131

1019. WHICH OF THE FOLLOWING AMINO ACIDS PROBABLY ACT AS STRONG EXCITATORY TRANSMITTERS?:

A. L-glutamate
B. Glycine
C. GABA
D. L-aspartate
E. Serine

Ref. 19 - p. 131

ANSWER THE FOLLOWING QUESTIONS (T)RUE OR (F)ALSE:

1020. Nervous tissue is capable of synthesizing pharmacologically active peptides. Ref. 19 - p. 135

1021. Subcellularly, substance P is located in brain tissue only as a bound form. Ref. 19 - p. 140

1022. Substance P preparations of brain tissue have been shown to consist of a family of related peptides. Ref. 19 - p. 141

1023. Nerve tissue extracts with substance P activity lose activity after incubation with chymotrypsin. Ref. 19 - p. 141

1024. Prostaglandins often antagonize the actions of adrenaline and noradrenaline. Ref. 19 - p. 150

1025. Prostaglandins are considered to be biologically active peptides. Ref. 19 - p. 151

1026. Prostaglandins are found only in nervous tissue. Ref. 19 - p. 156

1027. Prostaglandins are considered to be biologically active lipids.
Ref. 19 - p. 149

SELECT THE MOST APPROPRIATE ANSWER(S):

1028. WHICH OF THE FOLLOWING CHEMICAL MEDIATORS ARE LIBERATED AT POSTGANGLIONIC SYMPATHETIC NERVE ENDINGS UPON SWEAT GLANDS?:
A. Norepinephrine
B. Epinephrine
C. Acetylcholine
D. Substance P
E. Prostaglandins
Ref. 19 - p. 225

1029. WHICH OF THE FOLLOWING SUBSTANCES INHIBIT THE ACTION OF ACETYLCHOLINESTERASE?:
A. Atropine
B. Eserine
D. Neostigmine
D. Cholesterol
E. Estrogen
Ref. 19 - p. 225

1030. NERVE IMPULSES OF CHOLINERGIC FIBERS ARE CHARACTERISTIC OF WHICH OF THE FOLLOWING RESPONSES?:
A. Rapid
B. Diffuse
C. Localized
D. Slow
E. Short duration
Ref. 19 - p. 225

1031. WHICH OF THE FOLLOWING CELLS SHOW ONLY SLIGHT UPTAKE OF RNA PRECURSORS?:
A. Schwann cells
B. Oligodendrocytes
C. Astrocytes
D. Multipolar neurons
E. Betz cells
Ref. 20 - p. 44

1032. IN 1963, SHORE AND COLLEAGUES REPORTED THAT RESERPINE DEPLETED WHICH OF THE FOLLOWING?:
A. Dopamine
B. Dopa
C. Norepinephrine
D. Epinephrine
E. Serotonin
Ref. 20 - p. 63

1033. α-METHYLTYROSINE BLOCKS THE SYNTHESIS OF WHICH OF THE FOLLOWING?:
A. Dopa
B. Dopamine
C. Norepinephrine
D. 5-hydroxyindole acetic acid
E. Serotonin
Ref. 20 - p. 65

1034. THE MOST EFFECTIVE TREATMENT FOR DEPRESSION IN MAN INCLUDES WHICH OF THE FOLLOWING?:
A. Dehydroxyphenylserine
B. Reserpine
C. MAO inhibitors
D. Lithium salts
E. Electroconvulsive shock
Ref. 20 - p. 65

1035. WHICH OF THE FOLLOWING PREVENT THE ENZYMATIC DESTRUCTION OF ACETYLCHOLINE?:
A. Eserine
B. Nicotine
C. Muscarine
D. Cholinesterase
E. Hemicholinium
Ref. 21 - p. 78

1036. WHICH OF THE FOLLOWING ACT TO PREVENT THE RELEASE OF ACETYLCHOLINE?:
A. Clostridium botulinum
B. Calcium
C. Potassium
D. Tubocurarine
E. Dermacentor andersoni
Ref. 21 - pp. 82-83

1037. WHICH OF THE FOLLOWING ARE MUSCARINIC BLOCKING AGENTS?:
A. Tubocurarine
B. Atropine
C. Belladonna alkaloids
D. Scopolamine
E. Curariform drugs
Ref. 21 - p. 83

1038. WHICH OF THE FOLLOWING DRUGS AFFECT NICOTINIC SYNAPSES?:
A. Tubocurarine
B. Curariform drugs
C. Scopolamine
D. Belladonna alkaloids
E. Atropine
Ref. 21 - p. 83

1039. DOPA ENTERS THE STORAGE PARTICLES WHERE IT IS CONVERTED TO WHICH OF THE FOLLOWING?:
A. Serotonin
B. Acetylcholine
C. Norepinephrine
D. L-tyrosine
E. 5-hydroxytryptamine
Ref. 21 - p. 106

1040. IT APPEARS THAT THE PRIME ROLE OF __________ IS THE REGULATION OF THE INTRANEURONAL LEVEL OF CATECHOLAMINE:
A. Monoamine oxidase
B. Tyrosine hydroxylase
C. Calcium
D. Potassium
E. 5-hydroxytryptamine
Ref. 21 - p. 108

1041. THE HIGHEST CONCENTRATIONS OF DOPAMINE IN THE CENTRAL NERVOUS SYSTEM OCCUR IN WHICH OF THE FOLLOWING AREAS?:
A. Thalamus
B. Hypothalamus
C. Pineal
D. Caudate nucleus
E. Putamen
Ref. 21 - p. 109

1042. MOST OF THE CELL BODIES DEMONSTRATED TO CONTAIN NOREPINEPHRINE LIE IN WHICH OF THE FOLLOWING AREAS?:
A. Locus coeruleus
B. Reticular formation
C. Cortex
D. Insula
E. Pulvinar
Ref. 21 - p. 109

1043. CELL BODIES CONTAINING 5-HYDROXYTRYPTAMINE ARE LOCALIZED ALMOST EXCLUSIVELY TO WHICH OF THE FOLLOWING AREAS?:
A. Putamen
B. Globus pallidus
C. Claustrum
D. Amygdala
E. Raphe nuclei of brainstem
Ref. 21 - p. 109

1044. WHICH OF THE FOLLOWING ACT AS POSSIBLE TRANSMITTERS OF EXCITATION?:
A. Glutamate
B. GABA
C. Glycine
D. β-alanine
E. Amino-oxyacetic acid
Ref. 21 - p. 119

1045. WHICH OF THE FOLLOWING ACT AS POSSIBLE TRANSMITTERS OF INHIBITION?:
A. Glutamate
B. GABA
C. Glycine
D. β-alanine
E. Aspartate
Ref. 21 - p. 122

1046. WHICH OF THE FOLLOWING ARE THOUGHT TO IMPAIR LEARNING AND PERFORMANCE?:
A. Methylscopolamine
B. Methylatropine
C. Pentobarbital
D. Amphetamine
E. Atropine
Ref. 22 - p. 158

1047. WHICH OF THE FOLLOWING ARE THOUGHT TO FACILITATE LEARNING?:
A. Picrotoxin
B. Pentylenetetrazole
C. Strychnine
D. Atropine
E. Scopolamine
Ref. 22 - p. 185

1048. A FAILURE OF HYDROXYLATION OF PHENYLALANINE TO TYROSINE IN THE LIVER MAY RESULT IN WHICH OF THE FOLLOWING?:
A. Hartnup disease
B. Hepatolenticular disease
C. Phenylketonuria
D. Maple syrup disease
E. Wilson's disease
Ref. 22 - p. 198

1049. DISTURBANCES OF__________AND AMINO ACID METABOLISM ARE THE PREDOMINANT BIOCHEMICAL LESIONS IN WILSON'S DISEASE:
A. Iron
B. Copper
C. Potassium
D. Tryptophan
E. Phenylalanine
Ref. 22 - p. 202

1050. WHICH OF THE FOLLOWING DRUGS PRODUCE A THETA RHYTHM IN THE HIPPOCAMPUS?:
A. Anticholinesterases
B. Eserine
C. Diisopropylfluorophosphate
D. Atropine
E. Scopolamine
Ref. 22 - p. 94

1051. WHICH OF THE FOLLOWING DRUGS INHIBIT THE THETA RHYTHM IN THE HIPPOCAMPUS?:
A. Atropine
B. Scopolamine
C. Eserine
D. Pentobarbital
E. Anticholinesterases
Ref. 22 - p. 102

ANSWER THE FOLLOWING QUESTIONS (T)RUE OR (F)ALSE:

1052. No perivascular connective tissue sheath surrounds the CNS capillary.
Ref. 18 - p. 1

1053. Astrocytic and oligodendroglial processes completely invest the capillary basement membrane. Ref. 18 - p. 1

1054. Virchow-Robin spaces exist around capillaries. Ref. 18 - p. 1

1055. Experimental allergic encephalomyelitis is an example of a primary demyelinating disease. Ref. 18 - p. 11

1056. Electron microscopically, the first recognizable abnormality in allergic encephalomyelitis is swelling of astrocytes. Ref. 18 - p. 11

1057. It can be demonstrated that in cerebral edema there is a massive enlargement of the oligodendroglial cytoplasm. Ref. 18 - p. 17

1058. It can be demonstrated that in dehydration there is cytoplasmic contraction in oligodendrocytes. Ref. 18 - p. 17

1059. Injections of an antimetabolite of glucose (gold thioglucose) may specifically produce an oligodendroglial lesion in the hypothalamus. Ref. 18 - p. 20

1060. The pattern of glucose metabolism in cerebral tissue is similar to that in muscle, liver, adipose and other tissues. Ref. 18 - p. 27

1061. The utilization of fructose in cerebral tissue is much higher than that of glucose. Ref. 18 - p. 27

1062. The neurotropic drug, tofranil, suppresses the uptake of glycine into cerebral tissue. Ref. 18 - p. 66

1063. In maple syrup disease both the branched-chain amino acids, and branched-chain keto acids accumulate in the body. Ref. 18 - p. 74

1064. Phenylketonuria is due to a failure in phenylalanine hydroxylation. Ref. 18 - p. 83

1065. Large amounts of phenylalanine inhibit the uptake of tyrosine. Ref. 18 - p. 87

1066. According to prevailing concepts, membranes of animal cells are composed of a bimolecular leaflet of proteins in contact with layers of extended lipids. Ref. 18 - p. 159

1067. Chemical and enzymic investigations suggest that the process of myelin degeneration is the same in both the peripheral and central nervous system. Ref. 18 - p. 169

1068. Metachromatic leukoencephalopathy is a model of a genetically determined metabolic disorder affecting myelin. Ref. 18 - p. 214

1069. In metachromatic leukoencephalopathy excess metachromatic deposits occur only in the CNS. Ref. 18 - p. 214

1070. The main organic constituents of nervous tissue are proteins and lipoproteins. Ref. 18 - p. 268

SELECT THE MOST APPROPRIATE ANSWER(S):

1071. WHICH OF THE FOLLOWING AMINO ACIDS PASS THROUGH THE BLOOD BRAIN BARRIER TO BE RAPIDLY INCORPORATED INTO THE BRAIN PROTEINS?:

A. Tyrosine
B. Glutamic acid
C. Glycine
D. Methionine
E. Lysine

Ref. 18 - p. 271

1072. EXPERIMENTS BY AUTORADIOGRAPHIC METHODS HAVE SHOWN THAT METHIONINE-S^{35} ADMINISTERED IN VIVO IS INCORPORATED MAINLY IN PROTEINS OF WHICH OF THE FOLLOWING?:

A. Thalamus
B. Hypothalamus
C. Cingulate gyrus
D. Cerebellar cortex
E. Ammon's horn

Ref. 18 - p. 272

1073. THE BLOOD CAPILLARIES IN THE BRAINS OF ADULT MAMMALS HAVE PORES WHERE LARGE MOLECULES PENETRATE RELATIVELY QUICKLY IN WHICH OF THE FOLLOWING AREAS?:

A. Area postrema
B. Cerebellum
C. Neurohypophsis
D. Septum
E. Cingulate gyrus

Ref. 23 - p. 21

1074. UNCONJUGATED LIPIDS FOUND IN THE CNS INCLUDE WHICH OF THE FOLLOWING?:

A. Phospholipids
B. Cholesterol
C. Ester lipids
D. Desmosterol
E. Glycolipids

Ref. 23 - p. 49

1075. SOME ________ PERCENT OF THE CHOLESTEROL IN THE ADULT BRAIN IS LOCATED IN THE MYELIN SHEATH:

A. 20
B. 40
C. 30
D. 90
E. 70

Ref. 23 - p. 51

1076. THE MAJOR PHOSPHOSPHINGOLIPID IN ANIMAL TISSUES IS:

A. Sphingomyelin
B. Lecithin
C. Phosphorylcholine
D. Sphingosine
E. Cerebrosides

Ref. 23 - p. 51

1077. IN ADULT BRAIN UP TO 90% OF THE TOTAL CEREBROSIDES MAY BE PRESENT IN WHICH OF THE FOLLOWING?:

A. Dorsal root ganglion
B. Thalamus
C. Myelin sheath
D. Cerebellum
E. Mesencephalon

Ref. 23 - p. 51

1078. GANGLIOSIDES ARE CHARACTERISTICALLY FOUND IN WHICH OF THESE AREAS?:
A. Nerve endings
B. Internal capsule
C. Lateral funiculus
D. Grey matter
E. Posterior funiculus
Ref. 23 - p. 51

1079. WHICH OF THE FOLLOWING ARE CHARACTERISTIC OF BRAIN LIPOPROTEINS?:
A. Soluble in chloroform-methanol
B. Similar to plasma lipoproteins
C. Soluble in water
D. Insoluble in organic solvents
E. Insoluble in water
Ref. 23 - p. 56

1080. THE CONCENTRATION OF PROTEOLIPID PROTEIN IS ABOUT ______ TIMES HIGHER IN CENTRAL WHITE MATTER THAN IT IS IN GREY MATTER:
A. 70
B. 10
C. 20
D. 50
E. 5
Ref. 23 - p. 57

ANSWER THE FOLLOWING QUESTIONS (T)RUE OR (F)ALSE:

1081. 5-hydroxytryptophan is the precursor of 5-hydroxytryptamine.
Ref. 23 - p. 147

1082. 5-hydroxytryptamine is formed in other tissue and then migrates to the brain.
Ref. 23 - p. 148

1083. A small dose of 5-hydroxytryptophan produces depression and sedation.
Ref. 23 - p. 148

1084. In Parkinsonism the amount of dopamine in the relevant parts of the brain is lower than normal.
Ref. 23 - p. 150

1085. The amino acid histidine is the precursor of histamine.
Ref. 23 - p. 152

SELECT THE MOST APPROPRIATE ANSWER(S):

1086. 5-HYDROXYTRYPTAMINE, NORADRENALINE AND HISTAMINE ARE ALL CONCENTRATED IN WHICH OF THE FOLLOWING AREAS?:
A. Thalamus
B. Cerebral cortex
C. Hypothalamus
D. Area postrema
E. Caudate nucleus
Ref. 23 - p. 152

1087. LOWERING THE CONCENTRATION OF THE ENVIRONMENTAL GLUCOSE, EITHER IN VIVO OR IN VITRO, RESULTS IN AN INCREASE IN THE BRAIN LEVEL OF WHICH OF THE FOLLOWING?:
A. Alanine
B. Glycine
C. Glutamate
D. Aspartate
E. Glutamine
Ref. 23 - p. 155

ANSWER THE FOLLOWING QUESTION (T)RUE OR (F)ALSE:

1088. Both glutamate and aspartate are readily oxidized to carbon dioxide.
Ref. 23 - p. 156

SELECT THE MOST APPROPRIATE ANSWER:

1089. THE OXIDATION OF BOTH GLUTAMATE AND ASPARTATE MAY PRODUCE ABOUT__________% OF THE BRAIN RESPIRATORY CO_2:

A. 10
B. 80
C. 35
D. 5
E. 75

Ref. 23 - p. 156

ANSWER THE FOLLOWING QUESTIONS (T)RUE OR (F)ALSE:

1090. Phenylketonuria involves a deficiency of the enzyme phenylalanine hydroxylase. Ref. 23 - p. 159

1091. At least half of the lipid of the adult nervous system is present in myelin.
Ref. 23 - p. 191

1092. Triglycerides are found in high quantities within normal brain.
Ref. 23 - p. 194

1093. The central nervous system appears to depend almost exclusively on glucose as an energy source. Ref. 23 - p. 223

1094. Within the normal human range, there is a correlation between brain size and mental capacity or achievement.
Ref. 23 - p. 260

1095. In the adult brain, a relatively large fraction of glucose enters an amino acid pool before being oxidized to carbon dioxide.
Ref. 23 - p. 277

1096. High enzyme activity is associated with myelin.
Ref. 23 - p. 279

1097. During the process of myelination there are notable increases in enzyme activity. Ref. 23 - p. 279

1098. Histochemical examination shows that preceding myelination there is a marked increase in oxidative enzyme activity.
Ref. 23 - p. 279

1099. There are times during development when the embryonic brain is particularly vulnerable. Ref. 23 - p. 287

1100. One of the features of in vivo brain metabolism which distinguishes the brain from most other tissues is its great dependence on continuous supplies of oxygen and glucose. Ref. 23 - p. 290

SELECT THE MOST APPROPRIATE ANSWER(S):

1101. ________ARE VIRTUALLY DEVOID OF THE ENZYME CARBONIC ANHYDRASE:
A. Ependymal cells
B. Microglia
C. Astrocytes
D. Oligodendrocytes
E. Neurons
Ref. 23 - p. 333

1102. WHITE MATTER CONTAINS WHICH OF THE FOLLOWING?:
A. Neuronal perikarya
B. Axons
C. Dendrites
D. Oligodendroglia
E. Pyramidal cells
Ref. 23 - p. 334

1103. THE________IS OFTEN REGARDED AS THE "PUREST" GREY MATTER:
A. Thalamus
B. Hypothalamus
C. Subthalamus
D. Putamen
E. Caudate nucleus
Ref. 23 - p. 334

1104. GANGLIONIC GLIA ARE LOWER THAN THE NEURONS IN WHICH OF THE FOLLOWING ENZYMES?:
A. Hexokinase
B. Malate dehydrogenase
C. Glutamate dehydrogenase
D. Lactate dehydrogenase
E. Isocitric dehydrogenase
Ref. 23 - p. 343

1105. CYTOCHROME OXIDASE IS________PERCENT MORE ACTIVE IN NEURONS THAN IN GLIA:
A. 80
B. 20
C. 60
D. 40
E. 10
Ref. 23 - p. 343

1106. ________IS, WITH FEW EXCEPTIONS, THE ONLY PRACTICAL APPROACH TO THE STUDY OF THE CHEMICAL PATHOLOGY OF MENTAL ILLNESS IN LIVING HUMAN PATIENTS:
A. Isotopes
C. Brain biopsy
C. Body fluid analysis
D. Brain tissue aspirations
E. Brain fractionations
Ref. 23 - p. 377

1107. WHICH OF THE FOLLOWING APPEAR TO BE CHARACTERISTIC OF HUMAN MONOAMINE OXIDASE?:
A. Age dependency
B. Tissue specificity
C. Multiple forms
D. Same affinity for various substrates
E. Always elevated in brains of depressed patients
Ref. 24 - p. 18

1108. THE________OF TYROSINE TO DOPA IS CONSIDERED TO BE THE RATE-LIMITING STEP IN CATECHOLAMINE BIOSYNTHESIS:
A. Methylation
B. Oxidation
C. Amination
D. Hydroxylation
E. Reduction
Ref. 24 - p. 21

1109. TYROSINE HYDROXYLASE HAS BEEN ISOLATED FROM WHICH OF THE FOLLOWING TISSUES?:

A. Spleen
B. Pancreas
C. Adrenal cortex
D. Adrenal medulla
E. Brain

Ref. 24 - p. 21

1110. WHICH OF THE FOLLOWING STATEMENTS TEND TO BE ASSOCIATED WITH SCHIZOPHRENIC PATIENTS?:

A. React more commonly than normal with an acute psychosis to antabuse
B. Respond to phenothiazines and butyrophenones
C. Less reactive to histamine than normal people
D. Do not respond to LSD
E. Respond to methionine in all cases

Ref. 24 - p. 62

1111. ________ NONSPECIFICALLY INHIBITS THE ENZYME THAT CONVERTS DOPAMINE TO NORADRENALINE:

A. LSD
B. Methionine
C. Histamine
D. Phenothiazine
E. Antabuse

Ref. 24 - p. 62

1112. ________ INDIRECTLY DIMINISHES CATECHOLAMINE BIOSYNTHESIS BY INTERFERING WITH NOREPINEPHRINE BINDING:

A. Lithium
B. Reserpine
C. Alcohol
D. Imipramine
E. L-dopa

Ref. 24 - p. 80

ANSWER THE FOLLOWING QUESTIONS (T)RUE OR (F)ALSE:

1113. Cholesterol is the only sterol that occurs in appreciable amounts in adult nervous tissue. Ref. 23 - p. 50

1114. All the cholesterol present in the normal adult nervous system is in the free state. Ref. 23 - p. 50

1115. Esters of cholesterol do not occur in the adult nervous system. Ref. 23 - p. 51

1116. In the adult mammalian brain phospholipids account for 50 percent of the dry weight. Ref. 23 - p. 51

1117. Some 80 percent of the ethanolamine phospholipid in nervous tissue is in the form of the plasmalogen. Ref. 23 - p. 51

1118. Sphingomyelin accumulates in excessive amounts in the reticuloendothelial system of patients with Niemann-Pick's disease. Ref. 23 - p. 51

1119. Both cerebrosides and gangliosides belong to the classification of glycosphingolipids. Ref. 23 - p. 51

1120. Cerebrosides contain two molecules of hexose per molecule of cerebroside. Ref. 23 - p. 51

1121. Sulphatides are not normally found in the nervous system.
Ref. 23 - p. 51

1122. Gangliosides are hydrophilic as well as lipophilic.
Ref. 23 - p. 51

1123. Phosphoinositides are the lipids most closely associated with the protein in brain proteolipids. Ref. 23 - p. 56

1124. The concentration of proteolipid protein is about five times higher in central white matter than it is in grey matter.
Ref. 23 - p. 57

1125. The concentration of proteolipid protein in peripheral nerve is only about 10 percent of that in the white matter of the CNS.
Ref. 23 - p. 57

1126. There is evidence that the copper in the brain is bound to protein.
Ref. 23 - p. 58

1127. Multiple sclerosis is characterized neuropathologically by multiple focal lesions which show a predilection for white matter in the central nervous system. Ref. 23 - p. 74

1128. Amino acids of the brain are fairly inert.
Ref. 23 - p. 121

1129. Proteolipids have a relatively slow turnover in the brain.
Ref. 23 - p. 121

1130. During myelin formation the number of oligodendrocytes increases.
Ref. 18 - p. 10

1131. The formation of brain amino acids from the carbohydrates and pyruvate is strictly an aerobic process.
Ref. 18 - p. 27

1132. Low concentrations of tofranil suppress the uptake of glycine into cerebral tissue. Ref. 18 - p. 66

1133. The narcotic analgesic action of morphine is thought to relieve pain primarily by acting centrally. Ref. 26 - p. 97

1134. Aspirin is thought to block pain receptors in the periphery.
Ref. 23 - p. 97

SELECT THE MOST APPROPRIATE ANSWER(S):

1135. WHICH OF THE FOLLOWING ARE CHARACTERISTIC OF THE ACTION OF OPIUM ON THE NERVOUS SYSTEM?:
A. Depresses the central nervous system
B. Decreases the pain threshold
C. Causes a release of antidiuretic hormone
D. Induces euphoria
E. Retards all mental processes Ref. 25 - p. 103

1136. WHICH OF THE FOLLOWING ARE CHARACTERISTIC OF THE ACTION OF ASPIRIN ON THE NERVOUS SYSTEM?:
A. Antipyretic action
B. Vasodilation
C. Analgesic action
D. Addiction potential
E. Until modern times, the most important and extensively used of all drugs
Ref. 25 - p. 140

1137. WHICH OF THE FOLLOWING ARE CHARACTERISTIC OF THE ACTION OF BARBITURATES ON THE NERVOUS SYSTEM?:
A. Non-addictive
B. Exert little analgesic action
C. Induce sedation
D. Induce hypnotic effects
E. Usually induce euphoria
Ref. 25 - p. 159

1138. WHICH OF THE FOLLOWING DRUGS ARE USED IN TREATMENT OF THE CONVULSIVE STATES?:
A. Methadone
B. Noscapine
C. Codeine
D. Diphenylhydantoin
E. Phenobarbital
Ref. 25 - p. 182

1139. WHICH OF THE FOLLOWING DRUGS MAY BE CLASSIFIED AS STIMULANTS OF THE CENTRAL NERVOUS SYSTEM?:
A. Opium
B. Morphine
C. Codeine
D. Strychnine
E. Pentylenetetrazol
Ref. 25 - p. 146

1140. CAFFEINE CHARACTERISTICALLY INFLUENCES THE NERVOUS SYSTEM IN WHICH OF THE FOLLOWING WAYS?:
A. Potent sedative
B. Potent analgesic
C. Depression of the cortex
D. Controls convulsions
E. Stimulates the central nervous system
Ref. 25 - p. 201

1141. WHICH OF THE FOLLOWING DRUGS MIGHT BE CLASSIFIED AS PSYCHOTOMIMETIC AND PSYCHOTHERAPEUTIC?:
A. Chlorpromazine
B. Mepazine
C. Salicylates
D. Sulfinpyrazone
E. Thioridazine
Ref. 25 - p. 228

1142. WHICH OF THE FOLLOWING DRUGS ARE COMMONLY CLASSIFIED AS MINOR TRANQUILIZERS?:
A. Nikethamide
B. Equanil
C. Valium
D. Frenquel
E. Picrotin
Ref. 25 - p. 233

1143. WHICH OF THE FOLLOWING ARE CLASSIFIED AS ADRENERGIC DRUGS?:
A. Ephedrine
B. Amphetamine
C. Carbachol
D. Muscarine
E. Choline
Ref. 25 - p. 283

1144. WHICH OF THE FOLLOWING DRUGS COULD BE CLASSIFIED AS ALPHA-ADRENERGIC BLOCKING AGENTS?:

A. Azapetine
B. Bethanechol
C. Piperoxan
D. Acetylcholine
E. Tolazoline

Ref. 25 - p. 307

1145. WHICH OF THE FOLLOWING DRUGS COULD BE CLASSIFIED AS BETA-ADRENERGIC BLOCKING AGENTS?:

A. Pronethalol
B. Choline
C. Methacholine
D. Propranolol
E. Dichloroisoproterenol

Ref. 25 - p. 311

1146. WHICH OF THE FOLLOWING DRUGS COULD BE CLASSIFIED AS CHOLINERGIC DRUGS?:

A. Carbachol
B. Methacholine
C. Muscarine
D. Levophed bitrate
E. Syndrox

Ref. 25 - p. 317

1147. WHICH OF THE FOLLOWING WOULD BE CLASSIFIED AS ANTI-CHOLINERGIC DRUGS?:

A. Tolazoline
B. Azapetine
C. Tropane
D. Atropine
E. Scopine

Ref. 25 - p. 340

1148. WHICH OF THE FOLLOWING ACT ON AUTONOMIC GANGLIA?:

A. Caffeine
B. Nicotine
C. Tobacco
D. Nornicotine
E. Theophylline

Ref. 25 - p. 362

1149. WHICH OF THE FOLLOWING ACT AS GANGLIONIC BLOCKING AGENTS?:

A. Tetraethylammonium
B. Amitriptyline
C. Hexamethonium
D. Trimethaphan camsylate
E. Desipramine

Ref. 25 - p. 370

1150. WHICH OF THE FOLLOWING MIGHT BE CLASSIFIED AS NEURO-MUSCULAR BLOCKING AGENTS?:

A. Normetanephrine
B. Vanillyl mandelic acid
C. Decamethonium
D. Curare
E. Gallamine triethiodide

Ref. 25 - pp. 378, 380

ANSWER THE FOLLOWING QUESTIONS (T)RUE OR (F)ALSE:

1151. Edrophonium chloride exerts potent anticurare activity.

Ref. 25 - p. 382

1152. Analgesics are drugs which act on the nervous system to relieve pain and discomfort without dulling consciousness.

Ref. 25 - p. 96

1153. In general the analgesic drugs act by modifying pain receptors in the periphery. Ref. 25 - p. 97

1154. Morphine is the principal alkaloid of opium. Ref. 25 - p. 100

1155. Codeine has maintained its place as one of the most widely used analgesics since it only rarely produces addiction. Ref. 26 - p. 111

1156. Heroin acts more strongly on both cerebrum and medulla than does morphine. Ref. 25 - p. 114

1157. Barbiturates have a strong analgesic action and therefore are of great value in the presence of pain. Ref. 25 - p. 167

1158. The barbiturates are seldom used to suppress convulsions due to central nervous system stimulants. Ref. 25 - p. 168

1159. The barbiturates are used in psychiatric practice to induce hypnosis. Ref. 25 - p. 168

1160. The bromide ion exerts a stimulant action on the central nervous system. Ref. 25 - p. 168

1161. The anticonvulsants have the capacity to depress the motor activity of the central nervous system. Ref. 25 - p. 180

1162. Dilantin has made possible the management of convulsive seizures. Ref. 25 - p. 182

1163. Diphenylhydantoin is highly effective in patients with Petit Mal. Ref. 25 - p. 184

1164. Bemegride is used as a diagnostic aid in epilepsy. Ref. 25 - p. 197

1165. Nikethamide is used as an analeptic. Ref. 25 - p. 198

1166. Ritalin is a cortical stimulant which is more potent than amphetamine. Ref. 25 - p. 205

1167. Methylphenidate has been recommended as the drug of choice in the management of narcolepsy. Ref. 25 - p. 206

1168. The cerebellum contains about ten times as much acetylcholine as the rest of the brain. Ref. 25 - p. 211

1169. Serotonin is formed by decarboxylation of tryptophan to tryptamine which in turn is converted to serotonin by hydroxylation at C_5. Ref. 25 - p. 211

1170. In the presence of monoamine oxidase serotonin is oxidized to 5-hydroxyindole acetic acid. Ref. 25 - p. 212

1171. Serotonin is present in a concentration of approximately 0.5 mcg. per gram of brain tissue. Ref. 25 - p. 212

1172. Serotonin is highly concentrated in the cerebellum and only slightly concentrated in the hypothalamus. Ref. 25 - p. 212

1173. Serotonin contains an indole nucleus. Ref. 25 - p. 213

1174. Certain of the psychotomimetic drugs have been designated as psychedelic. Ref. 25 - p. 214

1175. Like alcohol, marihuana is a depressant. Ref. 25 - p. 218

1176. Unlike the barbiturates and other hypnotic agents, the tranquilizers act primarily on sub-cortical areas of the brain. Ref. 25 - p. 220

SELECT THE MOST APPROPRIATE ANSWER(S):

1177. THE MAJOR TRANQUILIZERS INCLUDE WHICH OF THE FOLLOWING?:
A. Chlorpromazine
B. Reserpine
C. Meprobamate
D. Diphenylmethane
E. Benzodiazepine
Ref. 25 - p. 220

1178. THE MINOR TRANQUILIZERS INCLUDE WHICH OF THE FOLLOWING?:
A. Propanediols
B. Diphenylmethane
C. Benzodiazepine
D. Reserpine
E. Chlorpromazine
Ref. 25 - p. 220

1179. WHICH OF THE FOLLOWING ARE DERIVED FROM THE RAUWOLFIA ALKALOIDS?:
A. Chloral hydrate
B. Paraldehyde
C. Petrichloral
D. Serpine
E. Reserpinine
Ref. 25 - p. 221

1180. MAJOR SITES OF ACTION IN THE BRAINS OF PATIENTS GIVEN PHENOTHIAZINES ARE THOUGHT TO INCLUDE WHICH OF THE FOLLOWING?:
A. Neocortex
B. Medulla
C. Hypothalamus
D. Reticular formation
E. Spinal cord
Ref. 25 - p. 223

1181. MAJOR SITES OF ACTION IN THE BRAINS OF PATIENTS GIVEN MEPROBAMATE ARE THOUGHT TO INCLUDE WHICH OF THE FOLLOWING?:
A. Reticular formation
B. Neocortex
C. Hypothalamus
D. Limbic system
E. Medulla
Ref. 25 - p. 223

ANSWER THE FOLLOWING QUESTIONS (T)RUE OR (F)ALSE:

1182. The action of reserpine on the autonomic centers includes depression of the sympathetic and facilitation of the parasympathetic centers in the diencephalon. Ref. 25 - p. 223

1183. Reserpine depletes histamine from the peripheral tissues.
Ref. 25 - p. 225

1184. The rauwolfia alkaloids potentiate the action of barbiturates and alcohol.
Ref. 25 - p. 225

1185. Reserpine also causes a depletion of the body stores of the adrenergic amines. Ref. 25 - p. 225

1186. Chlorpromazine stimulates the activity of the sympathetic nervous system. Ref. 25 - p. 228

1187. Patients most responsive to chlorpromazine are found to be suffering from a state of hallucinations and delusions of grandeur.
Ref. 25 - p. 229

1188. Patients suffering from a state of high arousal such as irritability, agitation and confusion are most responsive to fluphenazine.
Ref. 25 - p. 229

1189. Piperacetazide is an antidepressant. Ref. 25 - p. 229

1190. Chlorpromazine and promazine are effective in controlling the mania associated with alcoholic syndromes and the withdrawal of narcotics.
Ref. 25 - p. 230

1191. Haloperidol is used to treat agitated states associated with acute and chronic psychoses. Ref. 25 - p. 231

1192. Meprobamate acts primarily to block long internuncial circuits between the cortex and thalamus. Ref. 25 - p. 234

1193. Meprobamate is used widely to allay anxiety in psychoneurotics.
Ref. 25 - p. 234

1194. Drugs cause relaxation of skeletal muscle by acting on peripheral structures or by depressing subcortical and spinal synaptic transmission.
Ref. 25 - p. 235

1195. Valium is classified as a minor tranquilizer.
Ref. 25 - p. 236

1196. Librium is used widely in anxiety and tension.
Ref. 25 - p. 236

1197. MAO inhibitors exert a depressant action on the central nervous system.
Ref. 25 - p. 241

1198. Nardil is commonly used as an antidepressant.
Ref. 25 - p. 242

1199. The antidepressants most commonly used at present are the tricyclic iminodibenzyl derivatives and their metabolites.
Ref. 25 - p. 243

1200. Isoproterenol is unique among the sympathomimetic drugs in being an almost pure beta-adrenergic agonist devoid of alpha-adrenergic action.
Ref. 25 - p. 285

FOR EACH OF THE FOLLOWING MULTIPLE CHOICE QUESTIONS, SELECT THE MOST APPROPRIATE ANSWER(S):

1201. THE ARNOLD-CHIARI MALFORMATIONS ARE FREQUENTLY CHARACTERIZED BY THE FOLLOWING DISPLACEMENTS:
A. Cerebellar tonsils protrude into the spinal canal
B. Brain stem is stretched
C. Fourth ventricle is displaced caudally
D. Medulla is displaced to the middle cranial fossa
E. Third ventricle is displaced anteriorly
Ref. 8 - p. 77

1202. A FAILURE OF CLOSURE OF THE VERTEBRAE IS CALLED:
A. Papilledema
B. Spina bifida
C. Hydrocephalus
D. Meningocele
E. Platybasia
Ref. 8 - p. 76

1203. THE SYNDROME OF ANTERIOR SPINAL ARTERY THROMBOSIS INCLUDES WHICH OF THE FOLLOWING?:
A. Loss of pain and temperature sensibility below the involved cord segment
B. Partial loss of motor power below level of thrombosis
C. Complete loss of tactile sense and deep sensibility
D. Partial loss of conscious proprioception
E. A loss of motor power bilaterally in those muscles innervated by segments below the level of thrombosis
Ref. 8 - p. 113

1204. THE__________SYNDROME IS DUE TO HEMILATERAL COMMPRESSION OR TRANSECTION OF THE SPINAL CORD:
A. Anterior spinal artery
B. Brown-Séquard
C. Syringomyelia
D. Hematomyelia
E. Tabes dorsalis
Ref. 8 - p. 124

1205. A DISEASE CHARACTERIZED BY WIDESPREAD PATCHES OF DEMYELINATION WITH LESS PROMINENT AXIS CYLINDER DESTRUCTION AND GLIAL OVERGROWTH IS:
A. Syphilis
B. Poliomyelitis
C. Multiple sclerosis
D. Pernicious anemia
E. Amyotrophic lateral sclerosis
Ref. 8 - p. 126

1206. TABES DORSALIS CHARACTERISTICALLY INVOLVES WHICH OF THE FOLLOWING?:
A. Lateral spinothalamic pathway
B. Anterior gray column
C. Posterior roots
D. Corticospinal tracts
E. Posterior columns
Ref. 8 - p. 126

1207. WHICH OF THE FOLLOWING MAY BE CHARACTERISTIC OF SYRINGOMYELIA?:
A. Interruption of spinothalamic fibers
B. Cord cavitation
C. Dissociated sensory loss
D. Internuclear ophthalmoplegia
E. Hematomyelia — Ref. 8 - p. 125

1208. HORNER'S SYNDROME INCLUDES WHICH OF THE FOLLOWING?:
A. Ptosis of the upper eyelid
B. Loss of vibratory sense
C. Loss of sweating on the same side
D. Stereoanesthesia
E. Miosis of the pupil — Ref. 8 - p. 125

1209. HEMISECTION OF THE SPINAL CORD RESULTS IN WHICH OF THE FOLLOWING?:
A. Loss of position sense on opposite side
B. Impaired vibratory sense on the same side
C. Loss of pain and temperature sensation on same side
D. Impaired tactile discrimination on the opposite side
E. Level of sensory loss is usually not equivalent to that of the lesion but reaches several dermatomes below
Ref. 8 - p. 125

1210. IN HEART DISEASE, PAIN FREQUENTLY FELT DOWN INTO THE LEFT ARM AND HAND MAY BE RECOGNIZED AS:
A. Neuritis
B. Neuropathy
C. Myasthenia gravis
D. Raynaud's disease
E. Referred pain
Ref. 8 - p. 169

1211. NEOPLASMS COMPRISED OF GLIA CELLS (GLIOMAS) FORM ABOUT __________ OF ALL INTRACRANIAL TUMORS:
A. 10 to 20%
B. 40 to 50%
C. 50 to 65%
D. 75 to 95%
E. 3%
Ref. 10 - p. 32

1212. A LESION OF THE CROSSED SPINOTHALAMIC TRACT RESULTS IN THE LOSS OF __________ SENSE ON THE CONTRALATERAL SIDE OF THE BODY:
A. Touch and pressure
B. Conscious proprioceptive
C. Subconscious proprioceptive
D. Pain and temperature
E. Visceral pain — Ref. 6 - p. 142

1213. A LESION OF THE MEDIAL LEMNISCUS RESULTS IN WHICH OF THE FOLLOWING?:
A. Poor appreciation of shape and size
B. Loss of deep sensibility
C. Loss of pain and temperature sense
D. Astereognosis
E. Paraplegia — Ref. 6 - p. 142

1214. INTERRUPTION OF THE LATERAL LEMNISCUS RESULTS IN WHICH OF THE FOLLOWING?:
A. Total loss of audition
B. Loss of pain and temperature sense
C. Clonus
D. Paralysis
E. Diminution in audition Ref. 6 - p. 143

1215. IMPAIRMENT OF THE NUCLEUS AMBIGUUS AND ITS EFFERENT FIBERS RESULTS IN WHICH OF THE FOLLOWING?:
A. Dysphagia
B. Dysphonia
C. Dysarthria
D. Ptosis
E. Double vision
Ref. 6 - p. 143

1216. A FUNCTIONAL INTERRUPTION OF THE FACIAL NERVE RESULTS IN WHICH OF THE FOLLOWING?:
A. Partial paralysis of ipsilateral facial muscles
B. Loss of taste on one side of entire tongue
C. Inability to close the eyelid
D. Bell's palsy
E. Drooping of the side of the mouth Ref. 6 - p. 143

1217. DYSFUNCTION OF THE NEOCEREBELLUM RESULTS IN WHICH OF THE FOLLOWING?:
A. Hypotonia
B. Asthenia
C. Asynergia
D. Ataxia of the trunk muscles without signs of tremor or hypotonia
E. A tendency to fall backward, sway from side to side, and walk with a wide base Ref. 6 - pp. 152-153

1218. WHICH OF THE FOLLOWING SYMPTOMS ACCOMPANY CEREBELLAR DYSFUNCTION?:
A. Hypertonia
B. Terminal tremor
C. Adiadochokinesis
D. Hyperreflexia
E. Dysmetria
Ref. 6 - pp. 152-153

1219. VOLITIONAL MOVEMENTS OF THE EYE INVOLVE WHICH OF THE FOLLOWING CORTICAL AREAS?:
A. 6
B. 8
C. 19
D. 17
E. 41
Ref. 6 - p. 190

1220. THE COMPLETE INTERRUPTION OF THE OPTIC NERVE RESULTS IN WHICH OF THE FOLLOWING?:
A. Permanent blindness in one eye
B. Loss of accommodation in both eyes
C. Consensual light reflex remains intact in both eyes
D. Accomodation remains intact in both eyes
E. Scotoma Ref. 6 - p. 190

1221. A MIDLINE LESION OF THE OPTIC CHIASMA MAY RESULT IN WHICH OF THE FOLLOWING?:
A. Blindness in the nasal half of the retina
B. Blindness in the temporal half of the visual field of each eye
C. Bitemporal hemianopia
D. Loss of concensual light reflexes
E. Permanent blindness Ref. 6 - p. 190

1222. BILATERAL DAMAGE TO THE NONDECUSSATING FIBERS OF THE OPTIC CHIASMA RESULTS IN A:
A. Binasal hemianopia
B. Scotoma
C. Blindness in the temporal half of the retina
D. Loss of accommodation
E. Blindness in the nasal half of the visual field of each eye
Ref. 6 - p. 190

1223. THE COMPLETE INTERRUPTION OF THE OPTIC TRACT OR THE OPTIC RADIATIONS OR THE DESTRUCTION OF THE LATERAL GENICULATE BODY RESULTS IN WHICH OF THE FOLLOWING?:
A. Loss of accommodation
B. Contralateral homonymous hemianopia
C. Bitemporal hemianopia
D. Binasal hemianopia
E. Blindness in the field of vision on the opposite side of the lesion
Ref. 6 - p. 190

1224. IF AREA_________IS SEVERELY DAMAGED, A PATIENT IS UNABLE AUTOMATICALLY TO FOLLOW OBJECTS MOVING STEADILY ACROSS THE VISUAL FIELD OR TO SCAN A LINE OF PRINTED PAGE:
A. 4
B. 18
C. 6
D. 19
E. 3
Ref. 6 - p. 190

1225. INABILITY TO EXTEND THE ELBOW, WRIST, FINGERS AND THUMB OCCURS WITH INJURY TO WHICH OF THE FOLLOWING NERVES?:
A. Musculocutaneous
B. Radial
C. Median
D. Ulnar
E. Axillary
Ref. 7 - p. 208

1226. WRIST DROP IS THE MOST STRIKING FEATURE OF AN INJURY TO WHICH OF THE FOLLOWING NERVES?:
A. Axillary
B. Median
C. Ulnar
D. Musculocutaneous
E. Radial
Ref. 7 - p. 206

1227. THE MOST VULNERABLE POINTS OF THE_________NERVE ARE ITS BONY RELATIONS IN THE MIDDLE THIRD OF THE HUMERUS AND OVER THE LATERAL EPICONDYLE:
A. Median
B. Musculocutaneous
C. Radial
D. Axillary
E. Ulnar
Ref. 7 - p. 206

1228. THE WASTING OF THE THENAR EMINENCE AND THE ABNORMAL POSITION OF THE THUMB GIVE THE HAND A CHARACTERISTIC APPEARANCE AFTER_________ NERVE INJURY:

A. Median
B. Axillary
C. Ulnar
D. Radial
E. Musculocutaneous

Ref. 7 - p. 207

1229. THE__________NERVE IS PRONE TO TRAUMA AS IT CROSSES THE MEDIAL EPICONDYLE OF THE HUMERUS:

A. Ulnar
B. Median
C. Radial
D. Musculocutaneous
E. Axillary

Ref. 7 - p. 207

1230. INJURIES TO THE UPPER TRUNK OF THE BRACHIAL PLEXUS MAY BE ASSOCIATED WITH WHICH OF THE FOLLOWING?:

A. Syndrome of Klumpke
B. Syndrome of Duchenne-Erb
C. Involves muscles supplied by C5 and C6
D. Involves muscles of the hand
E. Difficulty in elevation and external rotation of the arm, accompanied by a severe loss of flexion and supination of the forearm

Ref. 7 - p. 208

1231. A LESION OF THE POSTERIOR CORD INVOLVES WHICH OF THE FOLLOWING NERVES?:

A. Radial
B. Axillary
C. Median
D. Ulnar
E. Musculocutaneous

Ref. 7 - p. 208

1232. INTERRUPTION OF THE LATERAL CORD AFFECTS WHICH OF THE FOLLOWING NERVES?:

A. Thoracodorsal
B. Subscapular
C. Musculocutaneous
D. Median
E. Ulnar

Ref. 7 - p. 208

1233. INJURY TO THE MEDIAL CORD INVOLVES WHICH OF THE FOLLOWING NERVES?:

A. Ulnar
B. Median
C. Medial brachial
D. Radial
E. Axillary

Ref. 7 - p. 208

1234. WHICH OF THE FOLLOWING STATEMENTS ARE RELATED TO INJURIES OF THE OBTURATOR NERVE?:

A. Abduction of the thigh is weakened
B. Sensory defects involve large area
C. Abduction of the thigh is completely lost
D. Inability to extend the leg
E. Abduction of the thigh is weakened

Ref. 7 - p. 209

1235. INJURY OF THE FEMORAL NERVE MAY CAUSE WHICH OF THE FOLLOWING?:
A. Inability to flex the leg
B. Relatively large areas of total anesthesia
C. Inability to adduct the thigh
D. Relatively no areas of anesthesia
E. Inability to extend the leg Ref. 7 - p. 209

1236. COMPLETE INTERRUPTION OF THE ________ NERVE ABOVE ALL ITS BRANCHES ABOLISHES PLANTAR FLEXION OF THE FOOT AND TOES AND SEVERELY IMPAIRS INVERSION OF THE FOOT:
A. Femoral
B. Obturator
C. Tibial
D. Lateral femoral cutaneous
E. Common peroneal Ref. 7 - p. 212

1237. WHICH OF THE FOLLOWING STATEMENTS APPLY TO TIBIAL NERVE INJURIES?:
A. Vulnerable to fractures of lateral malleolus
B. May be involved in the tarsal tunnel syndrome
C. Total anesthesia on the sole of the foot
D. Pes cavus
E. Paralysis of dorsal flexion Ref. 7 - p. 212

1238. COMPLETE SECTION OF THE PERONEAL NERVE CAUSES WHICH OF THE FOLLOWING?:
A. Paralysis of plantar flexion
B. Impairs inversion of the foot
C. Atrophy of the plantar muscles
D. Paralysis of dorsal flexion of the foot
E. Paralysis of eversion of the foot Ref. 7 - p. 212

1239. THE ________ NERVE IS SUBJECT TO INJURY BOTH BY COMPRESSION AND FRACTURE AT THE NECK OF THE FIBULA:
A. Femoral
B. Sciatic
C. Common peroneal
D. Tibial
E. Lateral plantar
Ref. 7 - p. 212

1240. WHICH OF THE FOLLOWING STATEMENTS MAY APPLY TO A TRAUMATIC NEUROMA?:
A. Consists of Schwann cells, macrophages and aberrant nerve fibers
B. May explain why a patient may have phantom pain
C. Cannot transmit impulses to the spinal cord
D. May be the cause of paresthesias
E. Contains no nerve fibers Ref. 7 - p. 214

1241. COMPLETE UNILATERAL DESTRUCTION OF THE VISUAL CORTEX IN MAN PRODUCES A:
A. Contralateral homonymous hemianopsia
B. Blindness in the ipsilateral nasal field
C. Blindness in the contralateral temporal field
D. Total blindness
E. Blindness in the contralateral nasal field
Ref. 7 - p. 562

1242. UNILATERAL LESIONS OF THE AUDITORY CORTEX CAUSE:
A. Total deafness
B. Partial deafness
C. A greater loss of hearing on the ipsilateral side
D. A greater loss of hearing on the contralateral side
E. No hearing deficits Ref. 7 - p. 567

1243. LESIONS OF AREA 22 IN THE DOMINANT HEMISPHERE CAUSE:
A. Word deafness
B. Loss of hearing
C. A loss in interpretation of sounds, especially speech
D. A form of sensory aphasia
E. Deficits in taste Ref. 7 - p. 568

1244. THE INABILITY TO PERFORM LEARNED SKILLED MOVEMENTS EVEN THOUGH NO PARALYSIS, SENSORY LOSS, OR ATAXIA IS PRESENT IS:
A. Tactile agnosia
B. Visual agnosia
C. Auditory agnosia
D. Apraxia
E. Aphasia
Ref. 7 - p. 585

1245. WHICH OF THE FOLLOWING STATEMENTS APPLY TO THE KLUVER-BUCY SYNDROME?:
A. Aggressive behavior
B. Docile behavior
C. Evidence of extreme fear
D. Psychic blindness
E. Bizarre sexual behavior Ref. 7 - p. 539

1246. DESTRUCTION OF WHICH OF THE FOLLOWING BRAIN AREAS IN THE DOMINANT HEMISPHERE USUALLY RESULTS IN "WORD BLINDNESS"?:
A. Area 37
B. Angular gyrus
C. Area 39
D. Superior temporal gyrus
E. Area 45 Ref. 9 - p. 515

1247. LESIONS IN WHICH OF THE FOLLOWING AREAS OF THE BRAIN CAUSE PATIENTS TO LOSE THE ABILITY TO USE WORDS AS A MEANS OF EXPRESSION OF THOUGHTS?:

A. Supramarginal gyrus
B. Area 3, 1 and 2
C. Area 40
D. Area 45
E. Premotor area

Ref. 9 - p. 515

1248. AN IMBALANCE IN THE ACTION OF TWO FUNCTIONING EYE MUSCLES, AGONIST AND ANTAGONIST, RESULTS IN WHICH OF THE FOLLOWING?:

A. Foville's syndrome
B. Progressive ophthalmoplegia
C. Weber's syndrome
D. Oculomotor ophthalmoplegia
E. Strabismus

Ref. 8 - p. 210

1249. A CAVERNOUS-SINUS THROMBOSIS MAY INVOLVE WHICH OF THE FOLLOWING?:

A. Oculomotor
B. Mandibular branch of trigeminal
C. Maxillary branch of trigeminal
B. Abducens
E. Trochlear

Ref. 8 - p. 211

1250. A UNILATERAL PARALYSIS OF THE EXTERNAL RECTUS AND A SEVERE PAIN IN THE SAME SIDE OF THE FACE, TOGETHER WITH SLIGHT SENSORY LOSS, MAY BE REFERRED TO AS__________ SYNDROME:

A. Gradenigo's
B. Millard-Gubler
C. Benedikt's
D. Weber's
E. Foville's

Ref. 8 - p. 211

1251. WHICH OF THE FOLLOWING MAY INVOLVE THE TRIGEMINAL NERVE?:

A. Bell's palsy
B. Geniculate neuralgia
C. Tic douloureux
D. Syringobulbia
E. Herpes zoster

Ref. 8 - pp. 216-217

1252. WHENEVER DISEASE DESTROYS THE FACIAL NUCLEUS OR INTERRUPTS THE COMPLETE FACIAL NERVE IN ITS PERIPHERAL COURSE, IT IS CUSTOMARY FOR THE FOLLOWING TO OCCUR:

A. Upper facial muscles are not completely paralyzed
B. The entire half of the face is paralyzed
C. Nodose neuralgia
D. Cardiac arrest with loss of consciousness
E. Convulsions

Ref. 8 - p. 222

1253. IN COMPLETE LESIONS OF THE VAGUS NERVE HIGH IN THE NECK, WE OBSERVE WHICH OF THE FOLLOWING?:
A. Ipsilateral paralysis of the levator veli palatine muscle
B. Contralateral paralysis of the constrictors of the pharynx
C. Contralateral paralysis of the tensor veli palatine muscle
D. Ipsilateral paralysis of the muscles of the larynx
E. Some awkwardness of swallowing Ref. 8 - p. 229

1254. BILATERAL VAGUS LESIONS MAY RESULT IN WHICH OF THE FOLLOWING?:
A. Dysphonia
B. Dysphagia
C. Bell's palsy
D. Glossal atrophy
E. Shingles
Ref. 8 - p. 229

1255. UNILATERAL NUCLEAR LESIONS OF THE SPINAL ACCESSORY NUCLEUS INCLUDE WHICH OF THE FOLLOWING?:
A. Paralysis of the trapezius muscle
B. Weakness of head rotation to opposite side
C. Inability to hold the head erect
D. Inability to raise the head from a recumbent position
E. Paralysis of the sternocleidomastoid muscle
Ref. 8 - p. 232

1256. A LOWER MOTOR NEURON HYPOGLOSSAL LESION INVOLVES WHICH OF THE FOLLOWING?:
A. Tongue muscle atrophy on opposite side of lesion
B. Protruded tongue deviates to the paralyzed side
C. Resting tongue deviates within the mouth toward the sound side
D. Tic douloureux
E. Pseudobulbar palsy Ref. 8 - p. 234

1257. THE SUDDEN OR RAPID LOSS OF ONE LABYRINTH CAUSES WHICH OF THE FOLLOWING?:
A. Vertigo
B. Nystagmus
C. Past pointing
D. Arnold-Chiari anomalies
E. Diplopia Ref. 8 - p. 254

1258. IN MENIERE'S "DISEASE" PATIENTS ARE PERIODICALLY SUBJECT TO WHICH OF THE FOLLOWING?:
A. Dysphonia
B. Vertigo
C. Nausea
D. Increased perspiration
E. Bell's palsy Ref. 8 - p. 254

1259. A MEDULLOBLASTOMA OF THE FLOCCULONODULAR LOBE OF THE CEREBELLUM CAUSES WHICH OF THE FOLLOWING?:
A. Gross defects of equilibrium
B. Flocculonodular syndrome
C. Hypotonia
D. Decreased reflexes
E. May be associated with increased intracranial pressure
Ref. 8 - p. 290

SECTION IV - NEUROPATHOLOGY AND CLINICAL PATHOLOGICAL CORRELATIONS

ANSWER THE FOLLOWING QUESTIONS (T)RUE OR (F)ALSE:

1260. Dysmetria denotes difficulty in gauging accurately the amount of movement necessary to attain an object.
Ref. 8 - p. 291

1261. Dysdiadochokinesis is the term for a disturbance of performing rapidly repetitive movement. Ref. 8 - p. 291

1262. In-coordination or awkwardness is commonly described as asthenia.
Ref. 8 - p. 292

1263. Cerebellar tremor usually increases near the termination of the movement. Ref. 8 - p. 292

1264. Diabetes insipidus occurs following the destruction of the supraoptic nuclei. Ref. 8 - p. 334

1265. Grand mal epilepsy characteristically shows a three-per-second spike-and-wave pattern from bilaterally synchronous foci.
Ref. 8 - p. 361

1266. Petit mal epilepsy does not appear to have a characteristic wave pattern associated with it. Ref. 8 - p. 361

1267. Increased muscle tone, hyper-reflexia, and clonus are signs of release and constitute spasticity. Ref. 8 - p. 390

1268. Convulsions recurring in an individual without known structural disease of the cortex, and in the absence of systemic disease, may be classed as idiopathic grand mal convulsions.
Ref. 8 - p. 393

1269. One of the most common diseases of the pyramidal motor system is paralysis agitans. Ref. 8 - p. 425

1270. In hepatolenticular degeneration severe disorder of muscle tone and a variety of involuntary movements, especially action tremors, are seen.
Ref. 8 - p. 425

1271. A generalized heightening in stretch reflex mechanisms, with widespread disorder of muscle tone which is clinically referred to as rigidity, is characteristic of diseases involving the basal ganglia.
Ref. 8 - p. 424

1272. Choreiform movements are rapid, jerky, and may appear to be somewhat purposive in character. Ref. 8 - p. 424

1273. Hemiballism is associated with destruction of the thalamus.
Ref. 8 - p. 426

1274. Huntington's chorea always occurs in children.
Ref. 8 - p. 426

SELECT THE MOST APPROPRIATE ANSWER(S):

1275. A PERSON WITH A LOSS OF TASTE IS SAID TO HAVE:
A. Parageusia
B. Hyposeusia
C. Ageusia
D. Gerstmann's syndrome
E. Ideomotor apraxia — Ref. 8 - p. 473

1276. TASTE HALLUCINATIONS MAY ARISE AS A FEATURE OF WHICH OF THE FOLLOWING AREAS?:
A. Insula
B. Uncus
C. Temporal lobe
D. Medulla
E. Area 6
Ref. 8 - p. 472

1277. COMPRESSION OF AN OPTIC NERVE WITHIN THE ORBIT OR WITHIN THE CRANIAL CAVITY MAY PRODUCE WHICH OF THE FOLLOWING?:
A. Atrophy of the nerve
B. Contralateral homonymous hemianopia
C. Heteronymous hemianopia
D. Bitemporal hemianopia
E. Varying degrees of visual defect — Ref. 8 - p. 501

1278. BITEMPORAL HEMIANOPIA OCCURS FOLLOWING LESIONS IN WHICH OF THE FOLLOWING AREAS?:
A. Compression of the chiasma from a lateral border
B. Compression of the crossing nasal retinal fibers
C. Injury of an optic nerve
D. Vascular lesions of the retina
E. Compression of the geniculocalcarine tract
Ref. 8 - p. 501

1279. THE FOSTER KENNEDY SYNDROME INCLUDES WHICH OF THE FOLLOWING?:
A. Homonymous hemianopia
B. Heteronymous hemianopia
C. Varying degrees of visual defect
D. Papilledema
E. Optic atrophy — Ref. 8 - p. 501

1280. HOMONYMOUS HEMIANOPIC DEFECTS WHICH DEVELOP SUDDENLY ARE MORE OFTEN DUE TO WHICH OF THE FOLLOWING?:
A. Vascular disorder
B. Trauma
C. Neoplasm
D. Degenerative disorder
E. Thrombosis — Ref. 8 - p. 502

1281. CHOREO-ATHETOID MOVEMENTS INCLUDE WHICH OF THE FOLLOWING TYPES OF MOVEMENT?:
A. Smooth
B. Irregular
C. Voluntary
D. Jerky
E. Involuntary
Ref. 12 - p. 424

1282. VIOLENT MOVEMENTS INVOLVING PROXIMAL PORTIONS OF THE EXTREMITY ARE CHARACTERISTIC OF WHICH OF THE FOLLOWING?:
A. Hemiballismus
B. Chorea
C. Athetosis
D. Tremor
E. Torsion spasm
Ref. 12 - p. 424

1283. WHICH OF THE FOLLOWING STATEMENTS APPLY TO THE TREMOR ASSOCIATED WITH PARKINSONISM?:
A. Abolished during ordinary movement
B. Abolished during sleep
C. Abolished by cutting the lateral corticospinal tract
D. Abolished by anterior chordotomy
E. Results from lesions of the cerebellum
Ref. 12 - p. 425

1284. RIGHT HOMONYMOUS HEMIANOPSIA MAY RESULT FROM LESIONS IN WHICH OF THE FOLLOWING AREAS?:
A. Right optic tract
B. Right geniculocalcarine fasciculus
C. Right optic nerve
D. Left optic tract
E. Left geniculocalcarine fasciculus
Ref. 12 - p. 430

1285. A BLINDNESS IN BOTH RIGHT UPPER QUADRANTS MAY RESULT FROM LESIONS IN WHICH OF THE FOLLOWING AREAS?:
A. Lower part of the left geniculocalcarine tract
B. Left optic nerve
C. Right optic tract
D. Optic chiasma
E. Lower part of the right geniculocalcarine tract
Ref. 12 - p. 430

1286. LESIONS INVOLVING THE __________ OR THE PATHS TO OR FROM IT MAY PREDISPOSE TO ULCERATION OR HEMORRHAGE IN THE ALIMENTARY TRACT:
A. Thalamus
B. Hippocampus
C. Hypothalamus
D. Epithalamus
E. Subthalamus
Ref. 12 - p. 311

1287. A DIRECT CONSEQUENCE OF A COMPLETE TRANSECTION OF THE SPINAL CORD AT UPPER CERVICAL LEVELS INCLUDES WHICH OF THE FOLLOWING?:
A. Spinal shock
B. Loss of all sensations below level of transection
C. Loss of voluntary control of motor activities below transection
D. Thermoregulatory mechanisms remain functional below level of transection
E. Permanent loss of reflexes below level of transection
Ref. 6 - p. 104

1288. HORIZONTAL DIPLOPIA ON LATERAL GAGE OCCURS IN LESIONS OF:
A. Abducens nerve
B. Facial nerve
C. Medial longitudinal fasciculus
D. Hypoglossal nerve
E. Oculosympathetic fibers Ref. 7 - p. 360

1289. THE MIDDLE ALTERNATING HEMIPLEGIA SYNDROME IS CHARACTERIZED BY WHICH OF THE FOLLOWING?:
A. Paralysis of the ipsilateral lateral rectus muscle
B. Ipsilateral hemiplegia
C. Contralateral hemiplegia
D. Lesions in the caudal pons
E. Paralysis of the contralateral superior oblique muscle
Ref. 7 - p. 361

ANSWER THE FOLLOWING QUESTIONS (T)RUE OR (F)ALSE:

1290. The inferior alternating hemiplegia involves the hypoglossal nerve and the medullary pyramid. Ref. 7 - p. 361

1291. Lesions of the spinal trigeminal tract result chiefly in loss or diminution of pain and thermal sense in the area innervated by the trigeminal nerve. Ref. 7 - p. 367

1292. Lesions involving the trochlear nerve alone are common and detection of resulting disturbances of extraocular movement is simple.
Ref. 7 - p. 378

1293. Lesions of the third nerve produce a contralateral lower motor neuron paralysis of the muscles supplied by the nerve.
Ref. 7 - p. 388

1294. Lesions of the third nerve produce external strabismus due to the unopposed action of the lateral rectus muscle.
Ref. 7 - p. 388

1295. A pupil which fails to constrict in bright light but responds to accommodation may be referred to as an Argyll-Robertson pupil.
Ref. 7 - p. 389

1296. Unilateral lesions of the mesencephalic tegmentum involving the red nucleus are described as producing a syndrome characterized by contralateral motor disturbances. Ref. 7 - p. 393

1297. Marked hypotonia associated with cerebellar disease may be related to interruption of afferent input from stretch receptors.
Ref. 7 - p. 434

1298. Cerebellar nystagmus is regarded as a fixation nystagmus.
Ref. 7 - p. 435

1299. Chorea appears to be the only form of dyskinesia resulting from a discrete lesion. Ref. 7 - p. 515

1300. Attempts to produce dyskinesia in experimental animals by creating lesions in the basal gnaglia have been highly successful.
Ref. 7 - p. 515

SELECT THE MOST APPROPRIATE ANSWER(S):

1301. WEBER'S SYNDROME IS CHARACTERIZED BY WHICH OF THE FOLLOWING?:
A. Lesion of the ventromedial midbrain
B. Contralateral ophthalmoplegia
C. Contralateral hemiplegia
D. Ipsilateral ophthalmoplegia
E. Associated with lesions of the quadrigeminal plate
Ref. 17 - p. 30

1302. WHICH OF THE FOLLOWING SYNDROMES ARE CHARACTERISTIC OF MIDBRAIN LESIONS?:
A. Turner's
B. Vail's
C. Benedikt's
D. Weber's
E. Parinaud's
Ref. 17 - p. 30

1303. WHICH OF THE FOLLOWING SYNDROMES ARE CHARACTERISTIC OF PONTINE LESIONS?:
A. Kleine-Levin
B. Millard-Gubler
C. Foville's
D. Raymond-Cestan
E. Korsakoff
Ref. 17 - p. 33

1304. THE HOMES-ADIE SYNDROME IS CHARACTERIZED BY:
A. A tonic pupillary reaction
B. Absence of one or more tendon reflexes
C. A pupil which has rapid contraction to light
D. Pupil which has rapid dilation upon removal of light stimulus
E. Abnormal blind spots in the field of vision.
Ref. 17 - pp. 91-92

1305. INJURY TO THE LONG THORACIC NERVE RESULTS IN WHICH OF THE FOLLOWING?:
A. Paralysis to the rhomboid muscles
B. "Winging" of the scapula
C. Difficulty in raising the arm above the horizontal
D. Paralysis of the serratus anterior
E. Claw-hand
Ref. 17 - p. 119

1306. CAUSALGIA IS CHARACTERIZED BY WHICH OF THE FOLLOWING?:
A. Painful sensations
B. Burning sensations
C. Nausea
D. Vesicular skin eruption
E. Anemia
Ref. 17 - p. 207

1307. ACROPARESTHESIA IS CHARACTERIZED BY WHICH OF THE FOLLOWING?:
A. Numbness and tingling sensations of fingertips
B. Trophic disorders of spinal cord
C. Numbness of toes
D. Scoliosis
E. Muscle paralysis Ref. 17 - p. 207

1308. GERSTMANN'S SYNDROME INCLUDES WHICH OF THE FOLLOWING?:
A. Disability in calculation
B. Finger agnosia
C. Writing disability
D. Usually associated with a focal lesion of the non-dominant cerebral hemisphere
E. Patient usually confabulates Ref. 17 - p. 227

1309. THE SCALENUS ANTICUS SYNDROME INCLUDES WHICH OF THE FOLLOWING?:
A. Pain in the chest
B. Atrophy of the small muscles of the hand
C. Numbness of the hand on the ulnar side
D. Pain in the arm, shoulder and neck
E. Platybasia Ref. 17 - p. 302

1310. HEPATOLENTICULAR DEGENERATION SHOWS WHICH OF THE FOLLOWING CHARACTERISTICS?:
A. Increase in copper excretion
B. Seldom fatal
C. Signs and symptoms of injury to the basal ganglia
D. Onset of symptoms is usually between the ages of 11 and 25 years
E. Optic atrophy and oculomotor palsies
Ref. 17 - p. 360

1311. THE HUTCHINSONIAN PUPIL IS CHARACTERIZED BY WHICH OF THE FOLLOWING?:
A. Pupil on the side of the lesion is first contracted and then widely dilated
B. Almost exclusively in females
C. Abnormality is unilateral in about 8 percent of cases
D. Pupil reacts to convergence but not to light
E. Atrophy of the iris Ref. 13 - p. 25

1312. WHICH OF THE FOLLOWING AREAS ARE MOST COMMONLY INVOLVED AS LESION SITES IN CONJUGATE OPHTHALMOPLEGIA?:
A. Medulla
B. Pons
C. Cerebellum
D. Thalamus
E. Caudate nucleus Ref. 13 - p. 30

1313. COMPLETE PARALYSIS OF THE THIRD CRANIAL NERVE RESULTS IN WHICH OF THE FOLLOWING?:
A. Complete ptosis of the upper lid
B. Constricted pupil
C. Pupil fails to react to light
D. Pupil reacts to accommodation
E. Paralysis of the medial rectus muscle
Ref. 13 - p. 31

1314. A FOURTH CRANIAL NERVE PARALYSIS RESULTS IN WHICH OF THE FOLLOWING?:
A. Partial ptosis
B. Weakness of the superior rectus muscle
C. Double vision when walking downstairs
D. Weakness of downward gaze
E. Loss of abduction of the eye
Ref. 13 - p. 31

1315. BOTH THE CORNEAL REFLEX AND JAW-JERK ARE MEDIATED BY WHICH OF THE FOLLOWING NERVES?:
A. Facial
B. Oculomotor
C. Trigeminal
D. Glossopharyngeal
E. Trochlear
Ref. 13 - p. 37

1316. A PATHOLOGICALLY EXAGGERATED JAW-JERK INDICATES WHICH OF THE FOLLOWING?:
A. Lower motor neuron lesion
B. Lesion below the level of the medulla
C. Upper motor neuron lesion
D. Lesion above the level of the pons
E. Seventh cranial nerve
Ref. 13 - p. 37

1317. WHICH OF THE FOLLOWING STATEMENTS APPLY TO MYELITIS?:
A. Inflammation of the corpus callosum
B. Involves only grey matter
C. Involves both grey and white matter
D. Inflammation of the spinal cord
E. May be due to the spread of bacterial infection
Ref. 13 - p. 274

ANSWER THE FOLLOWING QUESTIONS (T)RUE OR (F)ALSE:

1318. Encephaloceles are protrucions of the brain through anomalous clefts in the skull. Ref. 8 - p. 76

1319. The Babinski Reaction is considered to be an indication of injury to the lateral spinothalamic pathway. Ref. 8 - p. 122

1320. The Brown-Séquard Syndrome is due to bilateral compression or transection of the spinal cord. Ref. 8 - p. 124

1321. Tabes dorsalis characteristically first involves posterior roots and posterior columns. Ref. 8 - p. 126

1322. Argyll Robertson pupils are also frequently seen in tabes dorsalis. Ref. 8 - p. 126

1323. Multiple sclerosis is a disease characterized by widespread small patches of demylination, with a lesser degree of axis cylinder destruction, and glial proliferation. Ref. 8 - p. 126

1324. Amyotrophic lateral sclerosis is a degenerative disease which involves the posterior gray columns. Ref. 8 - p. 126

1325. Poliomyelitis characteristically involves the anterior and lateral intermediate gray columns of the spinal cord. Ref. 8 - p. 126

1326. Raynaud's Disease is a disorder of the basal ganglia. Ref. 8 - p. 126

1327. Projection of an image upon two asymmetric retinal foci will lead to the activation of asymmetric occipital lobe regions and result in the perception of two images of the object. Ref. 8 - p. 210

1328. When the oculomotor nerve is damaged with the peduncles, an ipsilateral oculomotor paralysis and a contralateral disturbance of motor power of the limbs result. Ref. 8 - p. 210

1329. Aneurysmal dilation of the superior cerebellar, posterior cerebral, or posterior communicating artery could compress either the oculomotor or trochlear nerve. Ref. 8 - p. 210

1330. A dilation of either the anterior inferior cerebellar or basilar artery might involve the abducens nerve. Ref. 8 - p. 210

1331. Herpes Zoster is infection, due to a virus, of motor neurons. Ref. 8 - p. 217

1332. The most common disorder of the facial nerve is the condition known as tic douloureux. Ref. 8 - p. 216

1333. In the majority of cases of Bell's Palsy, return of function gradually occurs. Ref. 8 - p. 223

1334. Unilateral lesions of the vagus are difficult to recognize. Ref. 8 - p. 229

1335. Syringomyelia is characterized by loss of pain and temperature sense in the affected parts. Ref. 16 - p. 207

1336. Lesions of the sensory parietal cortex usually impair the ability to recognize pain, temperature and vibration. Ref. 16 - p. 207

1337. Degeneration in the central nervous system differs from that in peripheral nerves in only one important respect. Ref. 15 - p. 397

1338. There is a well developed capillary network immediately beneath the pia.
Ref. 15 - p. 417

1339. Hippocampal herniation is related to the rigid tentorium lying between the middle and posterior fossae of the skull.
Ref. 15 - p. 426

1340. Cingulate herniation is related to the rigid falx which lies in the sagittal fissure between the hemispheres. Ref. 15 - p. 426

1341. Tonsillar herniations are related to the rigid tentorium.
Ref. 15 - p. 428

1342. The perivascular spaces (Virchow-Robin) are continuous with the subarachnoid space. Ref. 15 - p. 437

1343. The Queckenstedt test may be used to demonstrate that the spinal subarachnoid space is obstructed. Ref. 15 - p. 440

1344. Lumbar puncture is contraindicated if there are infections in skin or subcutaneous tissues, such as carbuncles or decubitus in the region of the puncture site. Ref. 15 - p. 448

1345. The Queckenstedt test should be performed in the presence of increased intracranial pressure. Ref. 15 - p. 448

1346. Obstructive hydrocephalus is most often the result of obstruction of the foramina of Monro or foramina of Magendie and Luschka rather than aqueductal stenosis. Ref. 15 - p. 459

1347. Astrocytes are the most vulnerable to toxic and anoxic conditions.
Ref. 15 - p. 541

1348. Astrocytic neoplasms are the most common primary tumors of the brain if the malignant forms are included.
Ref. 15 - p. 543

1349. The ganglioneuroma is a rapid growing tumor which is commonly found in the cerebellum. Ref. 15 - p. 578

SELECT THE MOST APPROPRIATE ANSWER(S):

1350. THE ALTERATION MOST OFTEN OBSERVED IN THE PINEAL BODY IS:
A. Cysts
B. Neoplastic changes
C. Calcification
D. Congenital defects
E. Hypoplasia
Ref. 15 - p. 614

1351. NEOPLASMS OF THE PINEAL BODY ACCOUNT FOR ________% OF ALL INTRACRANIAL NEOPLASMS:
A. 0.4-1
B. 4-11
C. 2-3
D. 12-21
E. 25
Ref. 15 - p. 614

1352. WHICH OF THE FOLLOWING SYMPTOMS MAY BE ASSOCIATED WITH PRIMARY TUMORS OF THE PINEAL BODY?:
A. Inability to turn the eyes upward
B. Ptosis
C. Constricted pupils
D. Argyll-Robertson pupils
E. Inability to move the eyes Ref. 15 - p. 614

1353. THE MOST CONSISTENT FINDING IN AMYOTROPHIC LATERAL SCLEROSIS IS THE INVOLVEMENT OF:
A. Basal ganglia
B. Cerebellum
C. Sensory cortex
D. Reticular formation
E. Anterior horn cells
Ref. 15 - p. 713

1354. WITH A LOWER MOTOR NEURON HYPOGLOSSAL LESION, THE TONGUE WOULD SHOW WHICH OF THE FOLLOWING?:
A. Atrophy on the paralyzed side
B. While at rest the tongue would be seen to be deviated within the mouth away from the sound side
C. When protruded the tongue would deviate to the paralyzed side
D. No atrophy
E. Small fascicular quiverings Ref. 8 - p. 234

1355. A JUGULAR FORAMEN SYNDROME WOULD INCLUDE WHICH OF THE FOLLOWING?:
A. Ptosis
B. Drooping of the shoulder
C. Nasal regurgitation of fluids
D. Dysphagia of solids
E. Paralysis of the tongue on the opposite side of the lesion
Ref. 8 - p. 234

1356. UPPER MOTOR NEURON PARALYSIS OF THE TONGUE INCLUDES WHICH OF THE FOLLOWING?:
A. Voluntary movements of the tongue are greatly impaired
B. Muscle atrophy
C. Speech is dysarthric
D. Fibrillations
E. Horner's Syndrome Ref. 8 - p. 235

1357. THE SUDDEN OR RAPID LOSS OF ONE LABYRINTH CAUSES WHICH OF THE FOLLOWING?:
A. Jugular foramen syndrome
B. Hoarseness
C. Vertigo
D. Nystagmus
E. Past pointing Ref. 8 - p. 254

1358. BILATERAL DESTRUCTION OF THE LABYRINTH PRODUCES WHICH OF THE FOLLOWING?:
A. Vertigo
B. Nystagmus
C. Disturbance of equilibrium
D. Pseudobulbar palsy
E. Torticollis — Ref. 8 - p. 254

1359. IRRITATIVE LESIONS OF THE MOTOR CENTERS OF THE CORTEX MAY CAUSE WHICH OF THE FOLLOWING?:
A. Convulsive seizures
B. Paralysis
C. Optic hallucinations
D. Acoustic hallucinations
E. Jacksonian epilepsy — Ref. 16 - p. 7

1360. DESTRUCTIVE LESIONS OF THE RIGHT MOTOR CORTEX (AREA 4) PRODUCE WHICH OF THE FOLLOWING?
A. Ipsilateral flaccid paresis of affected muscle group
B. Paralysis more pronounced in the distal portions of the extremities
C. Contralateral homonymous defects in the visual fields
D. Destruction of macular vision
E. Uncinate fits — Ref. 16 - p. 8

1361. SURGICAL PROCEDURES WHICH AFFECT THE CONNECTIONS BETWEEN THE FRONTAL CORTEX AND THE THALAMUS HAVE BEEN USED FOR WHICH OF THE FOLLOWING?:
A. Anxiety
B. Intractable pain
C. Astereognosis
D. Schizophrenic psychoses
E. Aphasia — Ref. 16 - p. 13

1362. LOSS OF RECENT MEMORY MAY OCCUR FOLLOWING EXTENSIVE BILATERAL_________LESIONS IN MAN:
A. Parietal lobe
B. Frontal lobe
C. Thalamic
D. Hippocampal
E. Lenticular
Ref. 16 - p. 15

1363. IN MAN, THERAPEUTIC PRODUCTION OF LESIONS OF THE_________ MAY REDUCE TREMOR AND RIGIDITY OF PATIENTS WITH PARKINSONISM OF DYSTONIA MUSCULORUM DEFORMANS:
A. Superior colliculate
B. Septum
C. Amygdala
D. Hippocampus
E. Globus pallidus
Ref. 16 - p. 17

1364. CLINICALLY IMPORTANT SYNDROMES CAUSED BY DYSFUNCTION OF THE_________SYSTEM MAY RESULT IN PARKINSONISM, ATHETOSIS, CHOREA AND TORSION SPASMS:
A. Limbic
B. Extrapyramidal
C. Pyramidal
D. Reticular
E. Ventricular
Ref. 16 - p. 17

1365. SOMNOLENCE MAY BE CAUSED REGULARLY BY BILATERAL LESIONS OF THE LATERAL_________AREA:
A. Amygdaloid
B. Septal
C. Thalamic
D. Hypothalamic
E. Hippocampal
Ref. 16 - p. 24

1366. IF THE_________NUCLEUS AND_________CORTEX ARE REMOVED BILATERALLY FROM A PLACID ANIMAL, A STATE OF FEROCITY FOLLOWS:
A. Septal, visual
B. Amygdaloid, pyriform
C. Caudate, auditory
D. Subthalamic, hippocampal
E. Thalamic, parietal
Ref. 16 - p. 24

1367. DESTRUCTION OF THE CORPORA QUADRIGEMINA CAUSES WHICH OF THE FOLLOWING?:
A. Paralysis of downward movements of the eye
B. Paralysis of upward movements of the eye
C. Spastic paralysis
D. Parinaud's Syndrome
E. Millard-Gubler Syndrome
Ref. 16 - p. 28

1368. WHICH OF THE FOLLOWING SYNDROMES MAY BE ASSOCIATED WITH MIDBRAIN LESIONS?:
A. Foville's
B. Millard-Gubler
C. Benedikt's
D. Parinaud's
E. Weber's
Ref. 16 - p. 30

1369. BEEVOR'S SIGN IS SEEN WITH SPINAL CORD LESIONS AT THE LEVEL OF THE_________SEGMENT:
A. First lumbar
B. Fifth cervical
C. Second sacral
D. Tenth thoracic
E. First cervical
Ref. 16 - p. 79

1370. THE FOSTER KENNEDY SYNDROME IS CHARACTERIZED BY WHICH OF THE FOLLOWING?:
A. Ipsilateral blindness
B. Ipsilateral anosmia
C. Myotonic pupils
D. Night blindness
E. Contralateral papilledema
Ref. 16 - p. 91

1371. ASTEREOGNOSIS IS THE LOSS OF:
A. Hearing
B. Vision
C. Taste
D. Ability to recognize objects owing to sensory impairment
E. Motor functions
Ref. 7 - p. 585

1372. WHICH OF THE FOLLOWING EYE PALSIES IS THE MOST COMMON?:
A. Abducens
B. Trochlear
C. Oculomotor
D. Ptosis
E. Graefe's disease
Ref. 16 - p. 96

1373. WHICH OF THE FOLLOWING SYMPTOMS MAY BE ASSOCIATED WITH DISORDERS OF THE TRIGEMINAL NERVE?:
A. Loss of jaw jerk
B. Loss of corneal reflexes
C. Impaired speech from paralysis of levator veli palatine muscle
D. Impaired hearing from paralysis of tensor tympani
E. Ptosis Ref. 16 - p. 99

1374. A LESION OF THE FACIAL NERVE OUTSIDE THE STYLOMASTOID FORAMEN WOULD INCLUDE WHICH OF THE FOLLOWING SYMPTOMS?:
A. Loss of taste in the anterior two-thirds of the tongue
B. Hyperacusis
C. Mouth droops
D. Food collects between cheeks and gums
E. Patient cannot close his eye Ref. 16 - p. 100

1375. A SUPRANUCLEAR TYPE OF FACIAL PALSY INCLUDES WHICH OF THE FOLLOWING?:
A. Flaccid type of paralysis
B. Taste and salivation are affected
C. Frontalis muscle is spared
D. Reaction of degeneration (RD) in facial muscles
E. Tonic spasm of muscles of mastication
Ref. 16 - p. 101

1376. CONSTRICTION OF THE POSTERIOR PHARYNGEAL WALL IN SAYING "AH" IS ABSENT WHEN THE__________NERVE IS INVOLVED:
A. Trigeminal
B. Facial
C. Vagus
D. Glossopharyngeal
E. Hypoglossal
Ref. 16 - p. 104

1377. THE PHARYNGEAL (GAG) REFLEX DEPENDS ON THE__________ NERVE FOR ITS SENSORY COMPONENT:
A. Ninth cranial
B. Eleventh cranial
C. Tenth cranial
D. Fifth cranial
E. Seventh cranial
Ref. 16 - p. 104

1378. WHICH OF THE FOLLOWING SYMPTOMS MAY BE SIGNS SUGGESTIVE OF TENTH CRANIAL NERVE INVOLVEMENT?:
A. Aphonia
B. Vertigo
C. Dysphonia
D. Nystagmus
E. Dysphagia
Ref. 16 - p. 106

1379. WHICH OF THE FOLLOWING SYMPTOMS MAY BE SIGNS SUGGESTIVE OF UNILATERAL PERIPHERAL INVOLVEMENT OF THE ELEVENTH CRANIAL NERVE?:
A. Atrophy of the affected sternocleidomastoid muscle
B. Cannot rotate head to healthy side
C. Spastic paralysis of the trapezius
D. Head drops forward
E. Cannot shrug affected shoulder Ref. 16 - p. 109

1380. WHICH OF THE FOLLOWING ARE CHARACTERISTIC OF KINETIC APRAXIA?:
A. Paresis
B. Cannot carry out automatic movements
C. May be confined to one limb
D. Expressive defect
E. Associated with lesions of the pre-central cortex
Ref. 7 - p. 587

1381. WHICH OF THE FOLLOWING ARE CHARACTERISTIC OF CONSTRUCTIONAL APRAXIA?:
A. Loss of visual guidance
B. Pure motor disorder
C. Inability to perceive spatial relationships
D. Paresis
E. Related to interruption of pathways between the occipital and parietal cortex
Ref. 7 - p. 587

1382. WHICH OF THE FOLLOWING SYMPTOMS MAY BE SIGNS OF PERIPHERAL INVOLVEMENT OF THE TWELFTH CRANIAL NERVE?:
A. Flaccid paralysis
B. Degeneration reaction
C. Contralateral paralysis of tongue
D. On protrusion the tongue deviates to the side of the lesion
E. No fibrillation or fasciculations of the tongue
Ref. 16 - p. 111

1383. VERNET'S SYNDROME (OF THE JUGULAR FORAMEN) USUALLY INVOLVES WHICH OF THE FOLLOWING NERVES?:
A. IX
B. X
C. VIII
D. XII
E. XI
Ref. 16 - p. 112

1384. JACKSON'S SYNDROME, PRODUCED BY A NUCLEAR OR RADICULAR LESION OF THE VAGUS, ACCESSORY AND HYPOGLOSSAL NERVES RESULTS IN WHICH OF THE FOLLOWING?:
A. Ipsilateral paralysis of the soft palate
B. Contralateral paralysis of the sternocleidomastoid muscle
C. Ipsilateral paralysis of the tongue
D. Atrophy of affected side of tongue
E. Contralateral paralysis of the trapezius muscles
Ref. 16 - p. 112

1385. A LESION OF THE PYRAMID NEAR THE DECUSSATION INVOLVING THE EMERGING HYPOGLOSSAL ROOTS WOULD SHOW WHICH OF THE FOLLOWING SYMPTOMS?:
A. Hypoglossal hemiplegia alternans
B. Contralateral hemiplegia
C. Contralateral Horner's Syndrome
D. Ipsilateral paralysis of the tongue
E. Ipsilateral loss of pain and temperature sense on the face
Ref. 16 - p. 112

1386. UNILATERAL PARALYSIS INVOLVING THE PHRENIC NERVE SHOWS WHICH OF THE FOLLOWING SYMPTOMS?:
A. Dyspnea
B. Short and rapid respiration
C. Fluoroscopy shows a relative immobility of diaphragm on one side
D. Litten's sign may be absent on the affected side
E. Liver or spleen may appear higher than normal
Ref. 16 - p. 118

1387. BILATERAL PARALYSIS INVOLVING THE PHRENIC NERVE SHOWS WHICH OF THE FOLLOWING?:
A. X-rays show the diaphragm drawn high into the chest
B. Dyspnea upon slightest exertion
C. Overactivity of accessory respiratory muscles
D. Few or no symptoms
E. Referred pain to the scrotal area Ref. 16 - p. 118

1388. PARALYSIS AND ATROPHY OF THE DELTOID, BICEPS, BRACHIALIS AND BRACHIORADIALIS MUSCLES WITH LOSS OF ABDUCTION AND EXTERNAL ROTATION OF THE ARM MAY BE CHARACTERISTIC OF WHICH OF THE FOLLOWING?:
A. Erb-Duchenne type injury
B. Klumpke type injury
C. Upper plexus type injury
D. Lower plexus type injury
E. Birth injury Ref. 16 - p. 118

1389. THE ARM AND HAND ASSUME THE "WAITER'S TIP" POSITION WITH WEAK FOREARM FLEXION AND SUPINATION IN WHICH OF THE FOLLOWING INJURIES TO THE BRACHIAL PLEXUS?:
A. Klumpke
B. Erb-Duchenne
C. Middle brachial plexus
D. Cervical nerves 7 and 8
E. Cervical nerves 5 and 6 Ref. 16 - p. 119

1390. A WINGED SCAPULA OCCURS FOLLOWING INJURIES TO WHICH OF THESE NERVES?:
A. Suprascapular
B. Long thoracic
C. Dorsal scapular
D. Thoracodorsal
E. Anterior thoracic
Ref. 16 - p. 119

1391. PARALYSIS OF THE CORACOBRACHIALIS, BICEPS AND BRACHIALIS MUSCLES OCCURS FOLLOWING INJURIES TO WHICH OF THESE NERVES?:
A. Medial brachial
B. Medial antebrachial cutaneous
C. Musculocutaneous
D. Thoracodorsal
E. Dorsal scapular Ref. 16 - p. 173

1392. THE INABILITY TO FLEX THE FOREARM WHEN IT IS SUPINATED, WEAKENED SUPINATION, LOSS OF BICEPS JERK AND ARM MUSCLE ATROPHY MAY OCCUR FOLLOWING COMPLETE PERIPHERAL INJURY TO WHICH OF THESE NERVES?:

A. Medial brachial
B. Thoracodorsal
C. Suprascapular
D. Dorsal scapular
E. Musculocutaneous

Ref. 16 - p. 123

1393. THE INABILITY TO PROTRACT OR RETRACT THE ARM OR RAISE IT TO THE HORIZONTAL POSITION OCCURS FOLLOWING INJURY TO WHICH OF THESE NERVES?:

A. Radial
B. Musculocutaneous
C. Thoracodorsal
D. Axillary
E. Medial brachial

Ref. 16 - p. 125

1394 WHICH OF THE FOLLOWING STATEMENTS ARE RELATED TO RADIAL NERVE INJURIES?:

A. Most commonly injured peripheral nerve
B. May be involved in both cervical cord and brachial plexus lesions
C. "Saturday Night Palsy"
D. Flexor paralysis
E. Inability to flex thumb

Ref. 16 - p. 125

1395. WHICH OF THE FOLLOWING STATEMENTS MAY BE APPLIED TO A COMPLETE RADIAL NERVE PALSY?:

A. Inability to extend the thumb
B. Supination of the hand with the wrist and fingers extended
C. Inability to make a fist
D. Triceps reflexes absent
E. Deltoid paralysis

Ref. 16 - p. 125

1396. WHICH OF THE FOLLOWING STATEMENTS MAY BE APPLIED TO A PERIPHERAL MEDIAN NERVE LESION?:

A. Wrist-drop
B. Muscle atrophy on dorsum of forearm
C. Thenar atrophy
D. Inability to oppose or flex the thumb
E. Weakened grip

Ref. 16 - p. 127

1397. WHICH OF THE FOLLOWING SYMPTOMS ARE ASSOCIATED WITH MEDIAN NERVE INJURIES?:

A. Loss of sensation over the distal phalanges of the first two fingers
B. Atrophy of the hypothenar eminence
C. Inability to flex the distal phalanx of the thumb
D. Flexion of fifth digit is weakened
E. Flexion of middle finger is weakened

Ref. 16 - p. 217

1398. WHICH OF THE FOLLOWING SYMPTOMS ARE ASSOCIATED WITH ULNAR NERVE INJURIES?:
A. Atrophy of the interosseous spaces
B. Claw hand
C. Inability to adduct the thumb
D. Atrophy of the thenar eminence
E. Triceps reflexes absent
Ref. 16 - p. 129

1399. A PATIENT IS UNABLE TO FLEX THE PROXIMAL OR DISTAL PHALANGES OF THE FOURTH AND FIFTH DIGITS FOLLOWING AN INJURY TO WHICH OF THESE NERVES?:
A. Radial
B. Median
C. Ulnar
D. Musculocutaneous
E. Axillary
Ref. 16 - p. 129

1400. WHEN THE AXON IS DIVIDED, DEGENERATIVE CHANGES PROGRESS:
A. Distally along the fiber for 2 or 3 cm from the site of injury
B. Distally the whole length of the axon
C. Centrally reaching the neuronal soma
D. Centrally and peripherally the whole length of the axon
E. 2 or 3 myelin segments in both directions
Ref. 7 - p. 139

1401. FOLLOWING SECTIONING OF THE PERIPHERAL NERVE ALL THE LISTED CHANGES OCCUR, EXCEPT:
A. Axonal degeneration distal to site of injury
B. Chromatolysis of cell body
C. Myelin degeneration distal to site of injury
D. Changes in neuronal organelles
E. Transsynaptic degeneration of adjacent neurons
Ref. 7 - p. 138

1402. REGENERATION IN THE PERIPHERAL NERVE INVOLVES ALL THE LISTED FUNCTIONS BELOW, EXCEPT:
A. Peripheral flow of axoplasm
B. Formation of Schwann cell tubes for the new axons
C. Formation of new myelin
D. Scar formation
E. Reinnervation of all the old sensory and motor endings
Ref. 7 - pp. 144, 215

1403. PAIN FROM A DISEASED DIAPHRAGM IS REFERRED TO DERMATOME:
A. C4
B. C8
C. T1 to 4
D. T6 to 9
E. T10 to 12
Ref. 7 - p. 189

1404. DURING NERVE REGENERATION AXONS GROW DISTALLY AT A RATE OF ________ A DAY:
A. 1-2 meters
B. 2-3 centimeters
C. 2-4 millimeters
D. 1-5 microns
E. 1-2 inches
Ref. 7 - p. 214

1405. PARALYSIS OF DORSAL FLEXION AND EVERSION OF THE FOOT AND LOSS OF DORSAL FLEXION OF THE TOES RESULTS FROM SECTIONING OF THE__________NERVE:
A. Femoral
B. Sciatic
C. Tibial
D. Common peroneal
E. Obturator
Ref. 7 - p. 212

1406. SECTION OF THE POSTGANGLIONIC NERVE FIBERS TO SMOOTH MUSCLE RESULTS IN:
A. Permanent flaccid paralysis
B. Failure to respond to circulating adrenalin
C. Degeneration of preganglionic fibers
D. Decreased sensitivity to adrenalin
E. Increased sensitivity to adrenalin Ref. 7 - p. 228

1407. LESION OF THE POSTERIOR COLUMNS PRODUCES THE FOLLOWING SYMPTOMS, EXCEPT:
A. Loss of two point discrimination
B. Poor tactile localization
C. Poor position sense of extremities
D. Poor movement sense of extremities
E. Loss of light touch Ref. 7 - p. 261

1408. UNILATERAL SECTION OF THE LATERAL SPINOTHALAMIC TRACT AT SPINAL SEGMENT T-1 PRODUCES:
A. Complete loss of pain and thermal sense on the same side of the body
B. Complete loss of pain and thermal sense of the viscera
C. Complete loss of pain and thermal sense on the opposite side of body extending to T-5 below the lesion
D. Complete loss of pain and thermal sense on the opposite side of body extending to T-2 below the lesion
E. Anesthesia of the superficial and deep portions of the body on the same side Ref. 8 - p. 125

1409. PARALYSIS OF BOTH LEGS IS KNOWN AS:
A. Monoplegia
B. Hemiplegia
C. Tetraplegia
D. Quadraplegia
E. Paraplegia
Ref. 7 - p. 280

1410. THE SYMPTOMS OF PYRAMIDAL LESION DO NOT INCLUDE:
A. Loss of volitional movement
B. Spasticity
C. Increased deep tendon reflexes
D. The sign of Babinski
E. Horner's syndrome Ref. 7 - p. 279

1411. THE SYMPTOMS OF LOWER MOTOR NEURON PARALYSIS DO NOT INCLUDE:
A. Degeneration of corticospinal fibers
B. Loss of all reflex movement
C. Loss of all voluntary movement
D. Loss of muscle tone
E. Rapid muscular atrophy Ref. 7 - p. 279

1412. LESION OF A VENTRAL ROOT C8 RESULTS IN:
A. Complete anesthesia in dermatome C7
B. No impairment in use of upper extremity
C. Paresis of the ipsilateral hand
D. Flaccid paralysis and atrophy of triceps brachii muscle
E. Spastic rigidity of triceps brachii muscle
Ref. 7 - p. 292

1413. INJURY TO THE DORSOLATERAL REGION OF THE MEDULLA MAY DESTROY BOTH THE SPINAL TRIGEMINAL TRACT AND THE SPINOTHALAMIC TRACT, PRODUCING LOSS OF PAIN AND TEMPERATURE:
A. On the same side of face and body
B. On the same side of face and the opposite side of the body
C. On the opposite side of face and body
D. On the opposite side of the face and same side of the body
E. On both sides of the body only Ref. 7 - p. 313

1414. AMYOTROPIC LATERAL SCLEROSIS IS CHARACTERIZED BY:
A. Progression of the disease over months to a few years
B. Progressive degeneration of the corticospinal tracts and anterior horn cells
C. Destruction of crossing fibers of the lateral spinothalamic tract
D. Loss of tactile, pressure and position sense on one side of the body
E. Loss of pain and temperature on both sides of the body
Ref. 7 - p. 292

1415. HEMISECTION OF THE SPINAL CORD (BROWN-SÉQUARD'S SYNDROME) PRODUCES ALL THE SYMPTOMS BELOW, EXCEPT:
A. Loss of sensory impulses in the posterior white columns below the lesion on the same side
B. Upper motor neuron lesion below the level of injury on the same side
C. Lower motor neuron symptoms and vasomotor paralysis on the side of the lesion at the level of injury
D. Loss of pain and thermal sense within the area of the lesion
E. Ipsilateral loss of pain and thermal sense below the level of the lesion on both sides Ref. 7 - p. 294

1416. INJURY TO THE MEDIAL LEMNISCUS CAUSES LOSS OF:
A. Pain and temperature sensation on the same side of the body
B. Pain and temperature sensation on the opposite side of the body
C. Kinesthetic and tactile sense on the same side of the body
D. Kinesthetic and tactile sense on the opposite side of the body
E. Auditory sensation on both sides of the body
Ref. 7 - p. 309

1417. MEDULLARY TRIGEMINAL TRACTOTOMY (INTERRUPTION OF THE SPINAL TRIGEMINAL TRACT) RESULTS IN:
A. Hyperactivity of mandibular reflexes
B. Increased tonus of the masticatory muscles
C. Loss of tactile sense
D. Loss of proprioceptive sense
E. Marked reduction in pain and thermal sense on the ipsilateral face
Ref. 7 - p. 313

1418. SYRINGOMYELIA WHICH EXTENDS INTO THE VENTRAL AND INTERMEDIOLATERAL GRAY OF SPINAL SEGMENTS C8-T1 PRODUCES ALL THE FOLLOWING SYMPTOMS, EXCEPT:
A. Increased threshold of two-point discrimination in the hands
B. Bilateral loss of pain and thermal sense in the distribution of spinal nerves and dermatomes (C8-T1)
C. Preservation of tactile, pressure and position sense
D. Lower motor neuron lesion
E. Horner's syndrome Ref. 7 - p. 292

1419. A LOWER MOTOR NEURON PARALYSIS OF THE IPSILATERAL HALF OF THE TONGUE AND A CONTRALATERAL HEMIPLEGIA RESULT FROM LESIONS OF:
A. Sensory-motor cortex near the lateral sulcus
B. Internal capsule at the genu
C. Lateral lemniscus
D. Pyramidal tract at the level of emerging root fibers of N. XII
E. One-half of spinal cord at upper cervical spinal level
Ref. 7 - p. 320

1420. UNILATERAL LESION OF THE VAGAL NERVE PRODUCES THE FOLLOWING SYMPTOMS OR SIGNS, EXCEPT:
A. Hoarseness
B. Dyspnea
C. Dysphagia
D. Elevation of soft palate on the normal side
E. Deviation of uvula to the side opposite the lesion
Ref. 7 - p. 324

1421. PSEUDOBULBAR PALSY (BILATERAL LESIONS OF CORTICOBULBAR FIBERS) PRODUCES A SYNDROME CHARACTERIZED BY THE FOLLOWING SYMPTOMS, EXCEPT:
A. Weakness of muscles which control swallowing and chewing
B. Weakness of muscles which control breathing and speaking
C. Little or no paralysis in the extremities
D. Loss of emotional control
E. Atrophy of muscles of face, tongue pharynx and larynx
Ref. 7 - p. 330

1422. UNILATERAL DESTRUCTION OF THE COCHLEAR NERVE OR BOTH COCHLEAR NUCLEI CAUSES:
A. Complete deafness on the same side
B. Complete deafness on the opposite side
C. Partial deafness on the opposite side
E. Loss of equilibrium Ref. 7 - p. 347

1423. LESION OF THE AUDITORY CORTEX CAUSES:
A. Complete loss of hearing on the same side
B. Complete loss of hearing on the opposite side
C. Bilateral diminution of hearing most marked in the contralateral ear
D. Complete loss of hearing in both ears
E. No disturbance in sound localization
Ref. 7 - p. 347

1424. CONDUCTION DEAFNESS RESULTS FROM THE LESION OF THE:
A. Ear ossicles
B. Cochlear nuclei
C. Superior olive
D. Inferior colliculus
E. Auditory sensory cortex Ref. 7 - p. 347

1425. ALL OF THE FOLLOWING STATEMENTS CONCERNING EFFECTS OF CENTRAL LESIONS INVOLVING CORTICOBULBAR AND CORTICORETICULAR FIBERS ON FACIAL NERVE FUNCTION ARE TRUE, EXCEPT:
A. Presence of marked weakness in the lower half of the face contralateral to the site of lesion
B. The muscles of the upper facial region manifest no weakness
C. The mimetic or emotional innervations of the facial muscles may be preserved
D. Flaccid paralysis of all muscles of expression
Ref. 7 - p. 360

1426. LESIONS OF THE ABDUCENS NERVE IN ITS INTRACRANIAL COURSE PRODUCE:
A. Contralateral paralysis of the lateral rectus muscle
B. Ipsilateral paralysis of the lateral rectus muscle
C. A strong abduction of the eye
D. Dropping of the superior eyelid Ref. 7 - p. 360

1427. TRIGEMINAL TRACTOTOMY OF THE SPINAL TRIGEMINAL TRACT CAN RELIEVE VARIOUS FORMS OF FACIAL PAIN WITHOUT IMPAIRING TACTILE SENSE. THE PROBABLE REASON FOR THIS IS THAT:
A. Tactile sense is not mediated by trigeminal nerve
B. Tactile and pressure sense reaches primarily the principal sensory nucleus of V
C. Tactile sense is mediated by a separate descending spinal trigeminal tract too diffuse to be cut surgically
D. Tactile stimulation from the face is carried primarily through cervical nerves of the cervical plexus
Ref. 7 - p. 368

1428. LESIONS OF THE THIRD NERVE PRODUCE ALL THE LISTED SYMPTOMS, WITH THE EXCEPTION OF:
A. External strabismus (squint)
B. Drooping of the eyelid (ptosis)
C. Dilation of the pupil (mydriasis)
D. Loss of pupillary light reflex and convergence
E. Loss of corneal reflex Ref. 7 - p. 388

1429. ALL OF THE LISTED SYMPTOMS RESULT FROM LESIONS OF THE CEREBELLAR HEMISPHERES (NEOCEREBELLUM), EXCEPT:
A. Flaccid paralysis
B. Dysmetria
C. Adiodochokinesis
D. Intentional tremor
E. Ataxia Ref. 7 - p. 434

1430. VASCULAR LESIONS IN THE POSTERIOR LIMB OF THE INTERNAL CAPSULE RESULT IN ALL THE LISTED SYMPTOMS, WITH THE EXCEPTION OF:
A. Contralateral hemianesthesia of the head
B. Contralateral hemianesthesia of the trunk
C. Contralateral hemianesthesia of the limbs
D. Contralateral hemiplegia
E. Unilateral hemianopsia Ref. 7 - p. 477

1431. BITEMPORAL HEMIANOPSIA RESULTS FROM A LESION OF THE:
A. Optic nerves
B. Optic chiasma
C. Optic tract
D. Lateral geniculate body
E. Primary visual cortex Ref. 7 - p. 482

1432. LESIONS OF THE THALAMUS PRODUCE SYMPTOMS LISTED BELOW, WITH THE EXCEPTION OF:
A. Disagreeable sensations
B. Loss of tactile localization
C. Loss of two-point discrimination
D. Loss of sense of position and movement
E. Hemiplegia Ref. 7 - p. 483

1433. HYPERPHAGIA RESULTS FROM BILATERAL LESIONS OF THE _________ HYPOTHALAMIC NUCLEUS:
A. Ventromedial
B. Dorsomedial
C. Anterior
D. Posterior
E. Lateral
Ref. 7 - p. 497

1434. SYMPTOMS ASSOCIATED WITH DISEASES OF THE EXTRAPYRAMIDAL SYSTEM DO NOT INCLUDE:
A. Tremor at rest
B. Athetosis
C. Chorea
D. Ballism
E. Agnosia Ref. 7 - p. 513

1435. IN PARALYSIS AGITANS, PATHOLOGICAL CHANGES ARE OBSERVED IN ALL THE LISTED STRUCTURES, EXCEPT THE:
A. Substantia nigra
B. Anterior horns of the spinal cord
C. Globus pallidus
D. Cerebral cortex
E. Brain stem reticular formation Ref. 7 - p. 515

1436. A LESION IN THE SUBTHALAMIC NUCLEUS IS USUALLY ASSOCIATED WITH:
A. Paralysis agitans
B. Athetosis
C. Ballism
D. Chorea
E. Huntington's chorea Ref. 7 - p. 515

1437. APHASIA MAY RESULT FROM A LARGE LESION INVOLVING THE:
A. Occipital lobe
B. Posterior temporoparietal region
C. Frontal pole
D. Temporal pole
E. Cerebellum Ref. 7 - p. 586

1438. KINETIC APRAXIA IS CHARACTERIZED BY INABILITY TO EXECUTE FINE MOTOR MOVEMENTS; THERE IS NO PARESIS, AND AUTOMATIC AND ASSOCIATED MOVEMENTS CAN BE CARRIED OUT. THE LESION MOST FREQUENTLY INVOLVES THE:
A. Postcentral cortex
B. Precentral cortex
C. Frontal lobe
D. Occipital lobe
E. Temporal lobe
Ref. 7 - p. 587

1439. WHICH OF THE FOLLOWING ARE CHARACTERISTIC OF AN ULNAR NERVE PARALYSIS?:
A. Patient is unable to flex the proximal or distal phalanges of the fourth and fifth digits
B. Fifth digit is adducted
C. Atrophy of the thenar eminence
D. Inability to adduct the thumb
E. Atrophy of the interosseous spaces Ref. 16 - p. 129

1440. WHICH OF THE FOLLOWING ARE CHARACTERISTIC OF A COMBINED MEDIAN AND ULNAR NERVE PARALYSIS?:
A. Loss of sensation on the radial side of the hand
B. The nail of the thumb may be deformed
C. Ulcerations may occur on the thumb
D. Atrophy of the thenar eminence
E. The patient cannot abduct or adduct the fingers
Ref. 16 - p. 130

1441. IF THE UMBILICUS MOVES UPWARD WHEN THE PATIENT TENSES HIS ABDOMEN (AS IN TRYING TO SIT UP FROM A RECLINING POSITION) IT IS KNOW AS:
A. Torsion spasm
B. Jacob syndrome
C. Beevor's sign
D. Vogt's sign
E. Leber's sign
Ref. 16 - p. 131

1442. WHICH OF THE FOLLOWING ARE CHARACTERISTIC OF LATERAL FEMORAL CUTANEOUS NERVE LESIONS?:
A. Meralgia paresthetica of Roth
B. Very common in young females
C. May occur as the first sign of a lumbar cord tumor
D. Numbness over the medial aspect of the thigh
E. Numbness and tingling, most marked on walking and standing
Ref. 16 - p. 133

1443. THE INABILITY TO EXTEND THE LEG AND LOSS OF KNEE JERK FOLLOWS AN INJURY TO WHICH OF THE FOLLOWING NERVES?:
A. Obturator
B. Femoral
C. Lateral femoral cutaneous
D. Sciatic
E. Sacral plexus
Ref. 16 - p. 135

1444. EXTERNAL ROTATION AND ADDUCTION OF THE THIGH ARE IMPAIRED FOLLOWING THE INJURY TO WHICH OF THE FOLLOWING NERVES?:
A. Obturator
B. Femoral
C. Sciatic
D. Lateral femoral cutaneous
E. Sacral
Ref. 16 - p. 135

1445. SECTION OF THE SUPERIOR GLUTEAL NERVE RESULTS IN WHICH OF THE FOLLOWING?:
A. Paralysis of the gluteus maximus
B. Paralysis of the gluteus medius
C. Weakened extensor power at the hip
D. Paralysis of the gluteus minimus
E. Weakened abduction of the leg
Ref. 16 - p. 137

1446. LOSS OF ACHILLES JERK AND PLANTAR REFLEX IS DUE TO AN INJURY OF THE__________NERVE:
A. Femoral
B. Obturator
C. Posterior femoral cutaneous
D. Sciatic
E. Inferior gluteal
Ref. 16 - p. 139

1447. PARALYSIS OF THE EXTENSOR-ABDUCTOR MUSCLES OF THE FOOT USUALLY OCCURS FOLLOWING INJURIES TO THE__________NERVE:
A. Femoral
B. Common peroneal
C. Obturator
D. Tibial
E. Superior gluteal
Ref. 16 - p. 141

1448. INABILITY TO PLANTAR-FLEX, ADDUCT, OR INVERT THE FOOT FOLLOWS AN INJURY TO THE__________NERVE:
A. Tibial
B. Common peroneal
C. Inferior gluteal
D. Femoral
E. Obturator
Ref. 16 - p. 143

1449. PARTIAL INCONTINENCE OF URINE AND FECES, TENESMUS AND DIFFICULTY ON URINATION MAY OCCUR FOLLOWING AN INJURY TO THE__________NERVE:
A. Superior gluteal
B. Obturator
C. Tibial
D. Pudendal
E. Sciatic
Ref. 16 - p. 144

1450. HORNER'S SYNDROME INCLUDES WHICH OF THE FOLLOWING?:
A. Ptosis
B. Miosis
C. Flushing of the face
D. Spinal shock
E. Megacolon
Ref. 16 - p. 155

ANSWER THE FOLLOWING QUESTIONS (T)RUE OR (F)ALSE:

1451. Hemiplegia is a paralysis of any two corresponding extremities. Ref. 16 - p. 168

1452. Hemiplegia alternans is a paralysis of one or more ipsilateral cranial nerves and contralateral paralysis of the arm and leg. Ref. 16 - p. 170

1453. In spasticity, there is increased resistance to sudden passive movements, and after the initial resistance there may be muscle relaxation. Ref. 16 - p. 171

1454. In rigidity, there is increased resistance on passive motion in any direction usually unrelated to speed or direction of movement. Ref. 16 - p. 171

1455. Hypotonia may occur with impaired muscle proprioceptive or motor innervation, cerebellar disease, or muscular disease. Ref. 16 - p. 171

1456. Psychogenic causes are the basis of many tics. Ref. 16 - p. 172

1457. Cerebellar tremors are commonly increased upon intention. Ref. 16 - p. 172

1458. Choreiform movements are usually due to an involvement of the cerebellum. Ref. 16 - p. 172

1459. Lesions of the cerebellum are characterized by continuous coordinated activity of the axial and proximal extremity musculature. Ref. 16 - p. 174

1460. Adiadokokinesia is the inability to perform rapidly alternating movements such as supination and pronation. Ref. 16 - p. 175

1461. Nystagmus is usually associated with extrapyramidal lesions. Ref. 16 - p. 175

1462. Plurosthotonus is the tendency to lean and fall to the side of the lesion.
Ref. 16 - p. 175

1463. Tabetic gait is characteristic of anterior horn cell disease.
Ref. 16 - p. 175

1464. Steppage gait occurs with paralysis of the anterior tibial group of muscles. Ref. 16 - p. 176

1465. Accoucheur's hand or "waiter's tip" position occurs with brachial plexus palsy. Ref. 16 - p. 176

1466. Sardonic smile is associated with facial muscle spasms of tetanus.
Ref. 16 - p. 176

1467. Posture in paralysis agitans is stooped with the head forward and elbows flexed. Ref. 16 - p. 176

1468. Causalgia is characterized by numbness and prickly or tingling sensations of the tips of the fingers and toes.
Ref. 16 - p. 207

1469. Herpes Zoster is due to a viral inflammation of the ventral root.
Ref. 16 - p. 207

1470. Tabes dorsalis is characterized by marked ataxia due to loss of the proprioceptive pathways. Ref. 16 - p. 207

1471. Syringomyelia is characterized by loss of pain and temperature sense with preservation of touch and pressure senses in the affected parts.
Ref. 16 - p. 207

1472. Advanced cases of pernicious anemia may be associated with combined degeneration of the posterior and lateral columns of the spinal cord.
Ref. 16 - p. 207

1473. Extension of the large toe with fanning of the small toes upon stimulation of the plantar surface of the foot is known as Babinski's sign.
Ref. 16 - p. 219

1474. Hyperactive reflexes occur with strychnine poisoning.
Ref. 16 - p. 219

SELECT THE MOST APPROPRIATE ANSWER(S):

1475. DYSMETRIA, WITH OVERSHOOTING OF THE MARK, IS OFTEN OBSERVED IN__________DISORDERS:

A. Thalamic
B. Hypothalamic
C. Cortical
D. Extrapyramidal
E. Cerebellar

Ref. 16 - p. 430

1476. IN DISORDERS CHARACTERIZED BY__________, AFFECTED MUSCLES MAY SHOW A PROLONGED RESPONSE TO SINGLE STIMULATION:
A. Jolly's myasthenia
B. Myotonia
C. Muscular dystrophy
D. Tetany
E. Familial periodic paralysis Ref. 16 - p. 256

1477. MENINGIOMAS USUALLY OBTAIN THEIR VASCULAR SUPPLY CHIEFLY FROM BRANCHES OF THE__________ARTERY:
A. Vertebral
B. Internal carotid
C. Maxillary
D. External carotid branches
E. Subclavian Ref. 16 - p. 268

1478. THE ABILITY TO HEAR A TUNING FORK BY AIR CONDUCTION IS COMPARED WITH THE ABILITY TO HEAR BY BONE CONDUCTION IN WHICH OF THE FOLLOWING TESTS?:
A. Schwabach's
B. Rinne's
C. Weber's
D. Bekesy's
E. Wickey's
Ref. 16 - p. 285

1479. IN DOWN'S SYNDROME, TRISOMY OF CHROMOSOME NO.__________ OCCURS, SO THAT THE TOTAL NUMBER OF CHROMOSOMES IS 47 INSTEAD OF THE NORMAL 46:
A. 7
B. 16
C. 21
D. 22
E. 3
Ref. 16 - p. 292

1480. WHICH OF THE FOLLOWING ABNORMALITIES MAY OCCUR WITH SPINA BIFIDA OCCULTA?:
A. Hypertrichosis
B. Telangiectases
C. Verbal amnesia
D. Motor aphasia
E. Disturbances in synergy Ref. 16 - p. 294

1481. IN THE DANDY-WALKER SYNDROME HYDROCEPHALUS IS CAUSED BY ATRESIA OF THE FORAMEN OF__________:
A. Luschka
B. Monro
C. Bethy
D. Magendie
E. Hyzenn
Ref. 16 - p. 297

1482. THE KLIPPEL-FEIL SYNDROME INCLUDES WHICH OF THE FOLLOWING?:
A. Reduction in cervical vertebrae
B. Hemangioblastomas of the cerebellum
C. Short neck
D. Cysts of the kidney
E. Limitation of motion of the neck Ref. 16 - p. 301

1483. OXYCEPHALY IS CHARACTERIZED BY WHICH OF THE FOLLOWING?:
A. Tumors of the skin
B. Hypertrophy of the tongue
C. Dome-shaped skull
D. Exophthalmos
E. Optic atrophy Ref. 16 - p. 300

1484. BRACHYCEPHALY RESULTS FROM PREMATURE CLOSURE OF THE ________ SUTURE:
A. Sagittal
B. Coronal
C. Intermaxillary
D. Lambdoidal
E. Temporozygomatic Ref. 16 - p. 300

1485. BABINSKI'S SIGN INCLUDES WHICH OF THE FOLLOWING?:
A. Extension of the large toe
B. Extension of the thumb
C. Fanning of the small toes
D. Loss of bladder and rectal reflexes
E. Loss of the light reflex Ref. 17 - p. 219

ANSWER THE FOLLOWING QUESTIONS (T)RUE OR (F)ALSE:

1486. Platybasia is a deformity of the occipital bone and upper end of the cervical spine. Ref. 16 - p. 302

1487. Intracerebral hemorrhage and thrombosis commonly occur in patients of 35 to 40 years of age. Ref. 16 - p. 304

1488. Occlusion of the main trunk of the posterior inferior cerebellar artery may cause ipsilateral facial analgesia. Ref. 16 - p. 313

1489. Occlusion of the superior cerebellar artery may cause contralateral ataxia. Ref. 16 - p. 313

1490. Occlusion of the basilar artery may cause flaccid quadriplegia. Ref. 16 - p. 313

1491. Cavernous sinus thrombophlebitis is usually secondary to suppuration in the orbit, nasal sinuses, or upper face. Ref. 16 - p. 323

1492. Acute infantile hemiplegia is believed to be due to inflammation of the branches of the posterior cerebral artery with resultant thrombosis and sensory involvement. Ref. 16 - p. 324

1493. Tabes dorsalis is a common syndrome associated with subdural abscesses. Ref. 16 - p. 325

1494. Romberg's sign is consistent with a loss of proprioceptive sense in the legs. Ref. 16 - p. 327

1495. Sydenham's chorea occurs in young individuals and is characterized by involuntary irregular movements, mild muscle weakness and, occasionally, mental disturbances. Ref. 16 - p. 332

1496. Medulloblastoma is a rapidly growing tumor of the medulla. Ref. 16 - p. 347

1497. Glioblastoma multiforme grow slowly and are usually found in the cerebellum. Ref. 16 - p. 347

1498. Spongioblastomas occur predominantly near the optic chiasm of children. Ref. 16 - p. 351

1499. Chromophobe tumors are relatively common in the posterior pituitary glands of adults. Ref. 16 - p. 351

1500. The average survival period of patients with spongioblastomas occurring in the brain stem is about one year. Ref. 16 - p. 351

1. Brodal, A.: Neurological Anatomy. Second Edition, Oxford University Press, New York, N.Y., 1969.

2. Bloom, W. and D. Fawcett: A Textbook of Histology. Ninth Edition, W.B. Saunders Co., Philadelphia, Pa., 1968.

3. Ham, A.: Histology. Sixth Edition, J.B. Lippincott Co., Philadelphia, Pa., 1969.

4. Greep, R.: Histology. Second Edition, McGraw-Hill Book Company, New York, N.Y., 1966.

5. Hamilton, W., J. Boyd and H. Mossman: Human Embryology. Third Edition, The Williams & Wilkins Company, Baltimore, Md., 1959

6. Noback, C.: The Human Nervous System. First Edition, McGraw-Hill Book Company, New York, N.Y., 1967.

7. Truex, R. and M. Carpenter: Human Neuroanatomy. Sixth Edition, The Williams & Wilkins Company, Baltimore, Md., 1969.

8. Peele, T.: The Neuroanatomic Basis for Clinical Neurology. Second Edition, McGraw-Hill Book Company, Inc., New York, N.Y., 1961.

9. Crosby, E., T. Humphrey and E. Lauer: Correlative Anatomy of the Nervous System. First Edition, The Macmillan Company, New York, N.Y., 1962.

10. Elliott, H.: Textbook of Neuroanatomy. Second Edition, J.B. Lippincott Co., Philadelphia, Pa., 1969.

11. Woodburne, R.: Essentials of Human Anatomy. Fourth Edition, Oxford University Press, New York, N.Y., 1969.

12. Ranson, S. and S. Clark: The Anatomy of the Nervous System. Tenth Edition, W.B. Saunders Company, Philadelphia, Pa., 1959.

13. Bannister, Roger: Brain's Clinical Neurology. Third Edition, Oxford University Press, New York, N.Y., 1969.

14. Brain, Lord and John Walton: Brain's Diseases of the Nervous System. Seventh Edition, Oxford University Press, New York, N.Y., 1969.

15. Minckler, Jeff, editor: Pathology of the Nervous System, Volume I. McGraw-Hill Book Company, New York, N.Y., 1968.

16. Chusid, Joseph G.: Correlative Neuroanatomy and Functional Neurology. Fourteenth Edition, Lange Medical Publications, Los Altos, California, 1970.

17. Ruch, T.C. and H.D. Patton: Physiology and Biophysics. Nineteenth Edition, W.B. Saunders Co., Philadelphia, Pa., 1965.

18. Korey, S., A. Pope and E. Robins: Ultrastructure and Metabolism of the Nervous System. The Williams & Wilkins Co., Baltimore, Md., 1962.

19. Lajtha, A.: Handbook of Neurochemistry, Volume IV. Plenum Press, New York, N.Y., 1970.

20. Cohen, M.M. and R.S. Snider: Morphological and Biochemical Correlates of Neural Activity. Harper & Row, Publishers, New York, N.Y., 1964.

21. McLennan, H.: Synaptic Transmission. W.B. Saunders Co., Philadelphia, Pa., 1970.

22. Pfeiffer, C. and J. Smythies: International Review of Neurobiology. Academic Press, New York, N.Y., 1965.

23. Davison, A. and J. Dobbing: Applied Neurochemistry. F.A. Davis Company, Philadelphia, Pa., 1968.

24. Ho, Beng T. and W.M. McIsaac. Brain Chemistry and Mental Disease. Plenum Press, New York, N.Y., 1971.

25. Grollman, A. and E. Grollman: Pharmacology and Therapeutics. Lea & Febiger, Philadelphia, Pa., 1970.

26. Guyton, A.C.: Textbook of Medical Physiology. Fourth Edition, W.B. Saunders Company, Philadelphia, Pa., 1971.

27. Tuttle, W.W. and B.A. Schottelius: Textbook of Physiology. Sixteenth Edition, The C.V. Mosby Company, Saint Louis, Mo., 1969.

ANSWER KEY

The authors have taken great pains to thoroughly check the questions and answers. However, in a volume of this size, some ambiguities and possible inaccuracies may appear. Therefore, if in doubt, consult your reference.

THE PUBLISHERS

SECTION I

1. C
2. D
3. B
4. E
5. D
6. A
7. B
8. E
9. C
10. A
11. E
12. B
13. D
14. C
15. E
16. C
17. E
18. D
19. D
20. D
21. E
22. E
23. E
24. A
25. D
26. A
27. C
28. E
29. A
30. E
31. D
32. A
33. A
34. E
35. E
36. E
37. E
38. C
39. A
40. E
41. E
42. A
43. B
44. E
45. D
46. E
47. A
48. C
49. E
50. D
51. E
52. C
53. C
54. C
55. E
56. C
57. B
58. B
59. A
60. C
61. E
62. C
63. C
64. D
65. E
66. A, C, E
67. A
68. B, E
69. E
70. A
71. A
72. C
73. E
74. E
75. C
76. A
77. A
78. E
79. A
80. B
81. E
82. B
83. C
84. A, B, E
85. E
86. D
87. C
88. C
89. C
90. D
91. C
92. B
93. B
94. E
95. B
96. D
97. A
98. A, B
99. C
100. B
101. D
102. E
103. E
104. C
105. C
106. D
107. E
108. A
109. E
110. A
111. B
112. E
113. A
114. B
115. E
116. C
117. E
118. E
119. E
120. A
121. B
122. E
123. E
124. B
125. C
126. B
127. C
128. E
129. D
130. D
131. C
132. A
133. B
134. C
135. C
136. A
137. C
138. D
139. C
140. E
141. C
142. C
143. B
144. E
145. E
146. D
147. D
148. A
149. B
150. B
151. B, D
152. E
153. E
154. D
155. D
156. C
157. A
158. A
159. D
160. D
161. C
162. E
163. E
164. D
165. E
166. A
167. D
168. C
169. A
170. E
171. D
172. B
173. E
174. E
175. B, C
176. B
177. E
178. C
179. B
180. D
181. A, C
182. A, B, E
183. C
184. A
185. B
186. A
187. E
188. C
189. D
190. C
191. D
192. B, C, D
193. C
194. E
195. B
196. C
197. C
198. C
199. E
200. E
201. C
202. A
203. D
204. C
205. B
206. B
207. C
208. A
209. D
210. E
211. C, D
212. A
213. E
214. E
215. D
216. D
217. E
218. A
219. E
220. E
221. A
222. E
223. E
224. E
225. D
226. E
227. A, B
228. A, B, C
229. B
230. A
231. B
232. D
233. C
234. B
235. D

236. D
237. E
238. B
239. E
240. A
241. C
242. A, B, E
243. E
244. B
245. A
246. C, D, E
247. B
248. D
249. E
250. B
251. E
252. D
253. E
254. B
255. E
256. D
257. B
258. E
259. D
260. A
261. E
262. A
263. B, D
264. C
265. B
266. A
267. D
268. E
269. E
270. A
271. D
272. D
273. A
274. D
275. E
276. B
277. D
278. D
279. E
280. C
281. B
282. D
283. E
284. E
285. A
286. C
287. D
288. A
289. E
290. A
291. A
292. B
293. C
294. B
295. C
296. E
297. B
298. A, C, E
299. E
300. A
301. A
302. A
303. D
304. E
305. E
306. D
307. E
308. D
309. B
310. A
311. C
312. A
313. A
314. B
315. A, B, C
316. B
317. E
318. D
319. A
320. A
321. B
322. E
323. C
324. D
325. D, E
326. E
327. B
328. B
329. A, C, E
330. C, E
331. C
332. E
333. C
334. C
335. E
336. B
337. C
338. E
339. A
340. D
341. E
342. E
343. E
344. C
345. A
346. D
347. A
348. B
349. D
350. B
351. E
352. D
353. A
354. B, C, D
355. A, C
356. B, C, D
357. A, E
358. B, C, E
359. C
360. C, E
361. B, D, E
362. A, B
363. A, B, C
364. A, C, E
365. E
366. A, E
367. C, D
368. C, D
369. C
370. A, B, C
371. A, D, E
372. A, C, E
373. A, C
374. A, D, E
375. C, E
376. C, D
377. D, E
378. B
379. A, E
380. B
381. A, B, E
382. C, D, E
383. A
384. E
385. C, E
386. A, C, D
387. B
388. A, B
389. D, E
390. A
391. F
392. T
393. T
394. T
395. F
396. T
397. F
398. T
399. T
400. T
401. B
402. C
403. E
404. E
405. A
406. D
407. D
408. B
409. B, C, E
410. A, C, E
411. B, D
412. A, E
413. B, D
414. D, E
415. B, C, E
416. C, D E
417. B, C
418. B, C, D
419. D, E
420. A, C
421. D
422. E
423. B, C
424. B, D
425. A, C
426. C, D
427. E
428. C
429. A, E
430. D
431. A, D, E
432. B, C
433. D
434. D
435. D
436. A
437. B
438. T
439. F
440. F
441. T
442. T
443. T
444. F
445. F
446. T
447. F
448. T
449. T
450. F
451. D
452. A
453. E
454. E
455. D

456. B
457. D
458. A
459. A
460. B
461. A, C, E
462. B, C, E
463. D
464. A
465. C, E
466. A, D, E
467. A, B, E
468. T
469. T
470. F
471. T
472. F
473. T
474. T
475. F
476. F
477. T
478. T
479. F
480. A, B
481. A, C, D
482. D, E
483. C
484. B, C, D
485. C, E
486. A, B, D
487. A, B
488. A, D
489. B, D
490. A, B, D
491. A, B
492. E
493. A, B
494. B, C, E
495. A, B, E
496. A, C, E
497. C, E
498. A, E
499. A, B, C
500. C, D
501. B, C, D
502. A, D, E
503. C, D
504. B, D, E
505. A, B, D
506. A, B, C
507. C, E
508. A, B, D
509. E
510. B, D, E
511. B, E
512. B, C, E
513. A, B
514. A, C
515. C, D
516. C, D
517. A, D, E
518. A
519. A, B, C
520. B, C, E
521. A, D, E
522. B, C
523. A, C, E
524. B, C
525. T
526. F
527. T
528. F
529. T
530. T
531. T
532. T
533. T
534. F
535. T
536. T
537. T
538. F
539. F
540. T
541. B
542. C
543. A, C
544. B, D
545. D
546. B, E
547. C, D
548. A, E
549. B
550. C, D
551. B, C, E
552. D
553. A, B, C
554. B, C, D
555. C, D, E
556. E
557. A
558. A, C, E
559. B
560. D
561. D
562. B, C
563. B, C, E
564. B
565. C
566. E
567. B
568. B, C, D
569. C, D, E
570. A, B, E
571. D
572. A
573. A, D, E
574. C
575. A
576. C
577. D
578. A, C, D
579. A, D
580. A, E
581. B, C, D
582. A, B, C
583. T
584. T
585. F
586. T
587. T
588. F
589. F
590. T
591. T
592. T
593. F
594. T
595. T
596. F
597. T
598. T
599. T
600. T
601. A
602. C, D, E
603. A, C, D
604. D
605. D
606. B, C
607. C
608. A, C, D
609. A, B, C
610. D
611. B, C, D
612. A
613. B, D
614. A, C, D
615. B, C, D
616. C, D
617. A, B, E
618. A, B, C
619. B
620. B, E
621. C, D, E
622. B, C
623. A, B
624. A, B, D
625. C
626. A
627. B
628. A, B, D
629. D
630. A, D
631. T
632. T
633. T
634. B, C, D
635. B, C, E
636. B, C
637. T
638. F
639. F
640. F
641. F
642. T
643. T
644. F
645. F
646. T
647. F
648. T
649. T
650. T
651. D
652. D, E
653. D
654. B, C
655. A, B
656. E
657. A, B, C
658. B, C, D
659. A, B
660. A, B
661. B, C, D
662 F
663. T
664. F
665. A, B, C
666. C
667. D
668. E
669. B
670. A, B
671. A, D
672. D
673. B
674. D, E
675. A, B, C

676. T
677. T
678. F
679. T
680. T
681. B
682. E
683. C, D, E
684. A, C, E
685. C
686. T
687. T
688. F
689. T
690. F
691. T
692. T
693. F
694. T
695. F
696. T
697. T
698. T
699. F
700. T

SECTION II

701. B
702. C
703. C
704. A
705. E
706. B
707. A
708. A
709. C
710. D
711. C
712. E
713. A
714. A
715. B
716. D
717. C
718. E
719. D
720. B
721. C
722. A
723. B
724. D
725. C
726. A
727. E
728. C
729. B
730. C
731. B
732. A
733. B
734. E
735. D
736. D
737. E
738. A
739. D
740. C
741. E
742. B
743. E
744. D
745. D
746. A
747. E
748. E
749. B
750. E
751. C
752. B
753. C
754. E
755. A
756. C
757. A
758. E
759. A
760. C
761. B
762. A
763. C
764. E
765. C
766. D
767. B
768. A
769. C
770. E
771. D
772. D
773. D
774. A
775. D
776. A
777. E
778. B
779. E
780. A
781. E
782. A
783. C
784. D
785. B
786. D
787. C
788. D
789. D
790. B
791. A
792. D
793. E
794. C
795. B
796. B
797. B
798. C
799. E
800. D
801. C
802. C
803. E
804. D
805. E
806. E
807. C
808. E
809. E
810. B
811. D
812. B
813. D
814. D
815. C
816. D
817. E
818. B
819. C
820. E
821. D
822. C
823. C
824. A
825. D
826. A
827. E
828. D
829. B
830. A
831. D
832. C
833. B
834. E
835. C
836. C
837. A
838. E
839. C
840. B
841. A
842. C
843. D
844. D
845. B
846. C
847. D
848. D
849. D
850. A
851. D
852. D
853. B
854. E
855. C
856. E
857. C
858. B
859. A
860. E
861. D
862. E
863. D
864. B
865. E
866. C
867. D
868. E
869. B
870. D
871. D
872. B
873. B
874. B
875. B
876. D
877. D
878. E
879. E
880. E
881. D
882. E
883. B
884. D
885. D
886. B
887. A
888. D
889. B
890. D
891. B
892. E
893. A
894. D
895. D
896. A
897. C
898. E
899. A
900. D
901. B
902. C
903. D
904. A
905. C
906. E
907. D
908. A
909. C
910. B
911. E
912. B
913. B
914. C
915. C
916. E
917. C
918. C
919. D
920. C
921. E
922. E
923. D
924. A
925. C
926. B
927. D
928. C
929. C
930. B
931. E
932. A
933. D
934. E
935. E
936. B
937. E
938. E
939. C
940. D
941. B
942. E
943. B
944. C
945. D
946. B
947. A

948. E
949. C
950. E
951. C
952. E
953. D
954. C
955. D
956. B
957. B
958. D
959. D
960. C
961. A
962. E
963. A
964. E
965. A
966. C
967. B
968. E
969. E
970. A
971. E
972. E
973. C
974. B
975. A, B
976. A, D
977. B, D
978. A, C, E
979. B, C
980. A, D, E
981. A, B, C
982. C, D
983. A, E
984. A, D
985. A, C
986. A, B
987. A, C, D
988. C, D
989. A, D
990. A, B, E
991. B, C, D
992. B, D, E
993. D, E
994. A, C, D, F, H
995. A, B, D
996. A, C, E
997. A, B, E
998. B, C, E
999. B, C

SECTION III

1000. D
1001. D
1002. A
1003. C
1004. C
1005. C, D
1006. A, B, E
1007. A
1008. B
1009. A, E
1010. A, D
1011. A, C
1012. A, D
1013. B
1014. C, D, E
1015. E
1016. E
1017. D
1018. B, C
1019. A
1020. T
1021. F
1022. T
1023. T
1024. T
1025. F
1026. F
1027. T
1028. C
1029. B, C
1030. A, C, E
1031. C
1032. E
1033. A, B, C
1034. E
1035. A
1036. A, E
1037. B, C, D
1038. A, B
1039. C
1040. A
1041. D, E
1042. A, B
1043. E
1044. A
1045. B, C, D
1046. C, D, E
1047. A, B, C
1048. C
1049. B
1050. A, B, C
1051. A, B, D
1052. T
1053. T
1054. F
1055. T
1056. F
1057. T
1058. T
1059. F
1060. F
1061. F
1062. T
1063. T
1064. T
1065. T
1066. F
1067. F
1068. T
1069. F
1070. T
1071. D, E
1072. D
1073. A, C
1074. B, D
1075. E
1076. A
1077. C
1078. A, D
1079. A, E
1080. E
1081. T
1082. F
1083. T
1084. T
1085. T
1086. C, D
1087. D
1088. T
1089. C
1090. T
1091. T
1092. F
1093. T
1094. F
1095. T
1096. F
1097. T
1098. T
1099. T
1100. T
1101. E
1102. B, C, D
1103. E
1104. A, B, C
1105. A
1106. C
1107. A, B, C
1108. D
1109. D, E
1110. A, B, C
1111. E
1112. B
1113. T
1114. T
1115. T
1116. F
1117. T
1118. T
1119. T
1120. F
1121. F
1122. T
1123. T
1124. T
1125. T
1126. T
1127. T
1128. F
1129. T
1130. T
1131. T
1132. T
1133. T
1134. T
1135. A, C, E
1136. A, B, C
1137. B, C, D
1138. D, E
1139. D, E
1140. E
1141. A, B, E
1142. B, C, D
1143. A, B
1144. A, C, E
1145. A, D, E
1146. A, B, C
1147. C, D, E
1148. B, C, D
1149. A, C, D
1150. C, D, E
1151. T
1152. T
1153. F

1154. T
1155. T
1156. T
1157. F
1158. F
1159. T
1160. F
1161. T
1162. T
1163. F
1164. T
1165. F
1166. F
1167. T
1168. F
1169. F
1170. T
1171. T
1172. F
1173. T
1174. T
1175. T
1176. T
1177. A, B
1178. A, B, C
1179. D, E
1180. C, D
1181. D
1182. T
1183. F
1184. T
1185. T
1186. F
1187. F
1188. F
1189. F
1190. T
1191. T
1192. T
1193. T
1194. T
1195. T
1196. T
1197. F
1198. T
1199. T
1200. T

SECTION IV

1201. A, B, C
1202. B
1203. A, E
1204. B
1205. C
1206. C, E
1207. A, B, C
1208. A, C, E
1209. B, E
1210. E
1211. C
1212. D
1213. A, B, D
1214. E
1215. A, B, C
1216. C, D, E
1217. A, B, C
1218. B, C, E
1219. B, C
1220. A, D
1221. A, B, C
1222. A, C, E
1223. B, E
1224. D
1225. B
1226. E
1227. C
1228. A
1229. A
1230. B, C, E
1231. A, B
1232. C, D
1233. A, B, C
1234. E
1235. B, E
1236. C
1237. B, C, D
1238. D, E
1239. C
1240. A, B,D
1241. A, B, C
1242. B, D
1243. A, C, D
1244. D
1245. A, D, E
1246. B, C
1247. A, C
1248. E
1249. A, D, E
1250. A
1251. C, D, E
1252. B
1253. A, D, E
1254. A, B
1255. A, B, E
1256. B, C
1257. A, B, C
1258. B, C, D
1259. A, B, E
1260. T
1261. T
1262. F
1263. T
1264. T
1265. F
1266. F
1267. T
1268. T
1269. F
1270. T
1271. T
1272. T
1273. F
1274. F
1275. C
1276. B, C
1277. A, E
1278. B
1279. C, D, E
1280. A, B, E
1281. B, D, E
1282. A
1283. A, B, C
1284. D, E
1285. A
1286. C
1287. A, B, C
1288. A, C
1289. A, C, D
1290. T
1291. T
1292. F
1293. F
1294. T
1295. T
1296. T
1297. T
1298. T
1299. F
1300. F
1301. A, C, D
1302. C, D, E
1303. B, C, D
1304. A, B
1305. B, C, D
1306. A, B
1307. A, C, D
1308. A, B, C
1309. B, C, D
1310. A, C, D
1311. A
1312. B
1313. A, C, E
1314. C, D
1315. C
1316. C, D
1317. C, D, E
1318. T
1319. F
1320. F
1321. T
1322. T
1323. T
1324. F
1325. T
1326. F
1327. T
1328. T
1329. T
1330. T
1331. F
1332. F
1333. T
1334. T
1335. T
1336. F
1337. T
1338. F
1339. T
1340. T
1341. F
1342. T
1343. T
1344. T
1345. F
1346. F
1347. F
1348. T
1349. F
1350. C
1351. A
1352. A, B, D
1353. E
1354. A, C, E
1355. B, C, D
1356. A, C
1357. C, D, E
1358. C
1359. A, B, E
1360. B
1361. A, B, D
1362. D
1363. E
1364. B
1365. D
1366. B
1367. B, D
1368. C, D, E
1369. D
1370. A, B, E

1371. D
1372. A
1373. A, B, D
1374. C, D, E
1375. C
1376. D
1377. A
1378. A, C, E
1379. A, B, E
1380. C, D, E
1381. A, C, E
1382. A, B, D
1383. A, B, E
1384. A, C, D
1385. A, B, D
1386. C, D, E
1387. A, B, C
1388. A, C, E
1389. B, E
1390. B
1391. C
1392. E
1393. D
1394. A, B, C
1395. A, C, D
1396. C, D, E
1397. A, C, E
1398. A, B, C
1399. C
1400. B
1401. E
1402. E
1403. A
1404. C
1405. D
1406. E
1407. E
1408. C
1409. E
1410. E
1411. A
1412. C
1413. B
1414. A, B
1415. E
1416. D
1417. E
1418. A
1419. D
1420. E
1421. E
1422. A
1423. C
1424. A
1425. D
1426. B
1427. B
1428. E
1429. A
1430. E
1431. B
1432. E
1433. A
1434. E
1435. B
1436. C
1437. B
1438. B
1439. A, D, E
1440. D, E
1441. C
1442. A, C, E
1443. B
1444. A
1445. B, D, E
1446. D
1447. B
1448. A
1449. D
1450. A, B, C
1451. F
1452. T
1453. T
1454. T
1455. T
1456. T
1457. T
1458. F
1459. F
1460. T
1461. F
1462. T
1463. F
1464. T
1465. T
1466. T
1467. T
1468. F
1469. F
1470. T
1471. T
1472. T
1473. T
1474. T
1475. E
1476. B
1477. C, D
1478. B
1479. C
1480. A, B
1481. D
1482. A, C, E
1483. C, D, E
1484. B
1485. A, C
1486. T
1487. F
1488. T
1489. F
1490. T
1491. T
1492. F
1493. F
1494. T
1495. T
1496. F
1497. F
1498. T
1499. F
1500. T

OTHER BOOKS AVAILABLE

ITEMS	Code	Unit Price
MEDICAL EXAM REVIEW BOOKS		
Vol. 1 Comprehensive	101	$12.00
Vol. 2 Clinical Medicine	102	7.50
Vol. 2A Txtbk. Study Guide of Int. Med.	123	7.50
Vol. 2B Txtbk. Study Guide of Int. Med.	130	7.50
Vol. 3 Basic Sciences	103	7.50
Vol. 4 Obstetrics-Gynecology	104	7.50
Vol. 4A Textbk. Study Guide of Gynecology	152	7.50
Vol. 5 Surgery	105	7.50
Vol. 5A Textbk. Study Guide of Surgery	150	7.50
Vol. 6 Public Health & Prev. Medicine	106	7.50
Vol. 8 Psychiatry & Neurology	108	7.50
Vol.11 Pediatrics	111	7.50
Vol.12 Anesthesiology	112	7.50
Vol.13 Orthopaedics	113	10.00
Vol.14 Urology	114	10.00
Vol.15 Ophthalmology	115	10.00
Vol.16 Otolaryngology	116	10.00
Vol.17 Radiology	117	10.00
Vol.18 Thoracic Surgery	118	10.00
Vol.19 Neurological Surgery	119	15.00
Vol.20 Physical Medicine	128	10.00
Vol.21 Dermatology	127	10.00
Vol.22 Gastroenterology	141	10.00
Vol.23 Child Psychiatry	126	10.00
Vol.24 Pulmonary Diseases	143	10.00
Vol.25 Nuclear Medicine	133	10.00
Vol.26 Allergy	132	10.00
Vol.27 Plastic Surgery	129	10.00
Vol.28 Cardiovascular Diseases	138	10.00
Vol.29 Oncology	146	10.00
ECFMG Exam Review - Part One	120	7.50
ECFMG Exam Review - Part Two	121	7.50
BASIC SCIENCE REVIEW BOOKS		
Anatomy Review	201	7.00
Biochemistry Review	202	7.00
Digestive System Basic Sciences	215	7.00
Heart & Vascular Systems Basic Sciences	212	7.00
Microbiology Review	203	7.00
Nervous System Basic Sciences	210	7.00
Pathology Review	204	7.00
Pharmacology Review	205	7.00
Physiology Review	206	7.00
Respiratory System Basic Sciences	213	7.00
Urinary System B.Sci.	214	7.00
Anatomy Textbook Study Guide	124	7.00
Histology Textbook Study Guide	151	7.00
Medical Physiology Textbk. Study Guide	155	7.00
SPECIALTY BOARD REVIEW BOOKS		
Dermatology Specialty Board Review	311	10.00
Family Practice Specialty Board Review	309	10.00
Internal Medicine Specialty Board Review	303	10.00
Neurology Specialty Board Review	306	10.00
Obstetrics-Gynecology Spec. Bd. Review	304	10.00
Pathology Specialty Board Review	305	10.00
Pediatrics Specialty Board Review	301	10.00
Psychiatry Specialty Board Review	312	10.00
Surgery Specialty Board Review	302	10.00
The Otolaryngology Boards	313	10.00

ITEMS	Code	Unit Price
The Psychiatry Boards	307	$8.00
STATE BOARD REVIEW BOOKS		
Med. State Brd. Rev.-Basic Sciences	411	9.00
Med. State Brd. Rev.-Clinical Sciences	412	9.00
Cardiopulmonary Techn. Exam. Rev.-Vol.1	473	7.50
Dental Exam. Review Book - Vol. 1	431	7.50
Dental Exam. Review Book - Vol. 2	432	7.50
Dental Exam. Review Book - Vol. 3	433	7.50
Dental Hygiene Exam. Review - Vol. 1	461	7.50
Emergency Med. Techn. Exam. Rev. - Vol.1	465	7.50
Emergency Med. Techn. Exam. Rev. - Vol.2	466	7.50
Immunology Exam. Review Book - Vol. 1	424	7.50
Inhalation Therapy Exam. Review - Vol. 1	471	7.50
Inhalation Therapy Exam. Review - Vol. 2	344	7.50
Laboratory Asst. Exam. Rev. Bk. - Vol. 1	455	7.50
Medical Librarian Exam. Rev. Bk. - Vol. 1	495	7.50
Medical Record Library Science - Vol. 1	496	7.50
Medical Techn. Exam. Review - Vol. 1	451	7.50
Medical Techn. Exam. Review - Vol. 2	452	7.50
Occupational Therapy Exam. Rev. - Vol.1	475	7.50
Optometry Exam. Review	469	10.00
Pharmacy Exam. Review Book - Vol. 1	421	7.50
Physical Therapy Exam. Review - Vol. 1	481	7.50
Physical Therapy Exam. Review - Vol. 2	482	7.50
X-Ray Technology Exam. Rev. - Vol. 1	441	7.50
X-Ray Technology Exam. Rev. - Vol. 2	442	7.50
X-Ray Technology Exam. Rev. - Vol. 3	443	7.50
NURSING EXAM REVIEW BOOKS		
Vol. 1 Medical-Surgical Nursing	501	4.50
Vol. 2 Psychiatric-Mental Health Nursing	502	4.50
Vol. 3 Maternal-Child Health Nursing	503	4.50
Vol. 4 Basic Sciences	504	4.50
Vol. 5 Anatomy and Physiology	505	4.50
Vol. 6 Pharmacology	506	4.50
Vol. 7 Microbiology	507	4.50
Vol. 8 Nutrition & Diet Therapy	508	4.50
Vol. 9 Community Health	509	4.50
Vol.10 History & Law of Nursing	510	4.50
Vol.11 Fundamentals of Nursing	511	4.50
Practical Nursing Examination Rev.-Vol.1	711	4.50
CASE STUDY BOOKS		
Allergy Case Studies	027	10.00
Cardiology Case Studies	001	10.00
Chest Diseases Case Studies	012	10.00
Child Psychiatry Case Studies	029	10.00
Cutaneous Medicine Case Studies	014	7.50
ECG Case Studies	003	7.50
Endocrinology Case Studies	008	10.00
Gastroenterology Case Studies	004	10.00
Hematology Case Studies	020	10.00
Infectious Diseases Case Studies	011	7.50
Neurology Case Studies	006	10.00
Otolaryngology Case Studies	021	10.00
Pediatric Hematology Case Studies	018	10.00
Pediatric Oculo-Neural Dis. Case Studies	023	10.00
Respiratory Care Case Studies	019	7.50
Urology Case Studies	017	10.00
MEDICAL OUTLINE SERIES		
Cancer Chemotherapy	631	10.00
Child Psychiatry	613	10.00

Prices subject to change.

OTHER BOOKS AVAILABLE

ITEMS	Code	Unit Price
MEDICAL OUTLINE SERIES *(Cont'd.)*		
Endocrinology	614	$10.00
Histology	662	8.00
Otolaryngology	661	8.00
Psychiatry	621	8.00
Urology	611	8.00
SELF-ASSESSMENT BOOKS		
Self-Assess. Cur. Knldge - Biochemistry	266	7.50
S.A.C.K. in Cardiovascular Diseases	275	10.00
S.A.C.K. in Family Practice	261	10.00
S.A.C.K. in Infectious Diseases	263	10.00
S.A.C.K. in Internal Medicine	257	10.00
S.A.C.K. in Neurology	254	10.00
S.A.C.K. for Nurse Anesthetist	715	7.50
S.A.C.K. in O.R. Techn.	474	7.50
S.A.C.K. in Otolaryngology	270	10.00
S.A.C.K. in Pathology	253	10.00
S.A.C.K. in Pediatrics	256	10.00
S.A.C.K. in Psychiatry	252	10.00
S.A.C.K. in Pulmonary Diseases	271	10.00
S.A.C.K. in Rheumatology	258	10.00
S.A.C.K. in Surgery	250	10.00
S.A.C.K. in Surgery for Family Physicians	259	10.00
S.A.C.K. in Urology	251	10.00
MEDICAL HANDBOOKS		
Medical Emergencies	635	8.00
Neurology	604	8.00
Obstetrical Emergencies	634	8.00
Ophthalmologic Emergencies	633	8.00
Pediatric Anesthesia	637	8.00
Pediatric Neurology	636	10.00
PRACTICAL POINTS BOOKS		
In Anesthesiology	700	10.00
In Gastroenterology	733	7.00
In Pediatrics	702	10.00
PRACTITIONERS GUIDES		
OB-Gynecology Disorders	704	10.00
Ophthalmologic Disorders	703	10.00
JOURNAL ARTICLE COMPILATIONS		
Ambulance Service Journal Articles	517	10.00
Blood Banking & Immunohemat. Jour. Art.	798	10.00
Emergency Room Journal Articles	795	8.00
Hodgkin's Disease Journal Articles	515	12.00
Hosp. & Inst. Eng. & Maintenance J. Art.	793	8.00
Hosp. Electronic Data Process. J. Art.	791	8.00
Hosp. Pharmacy Journal Articles	799	10.00
Hosp. Security & Safety Journal Articles	796	8.00
Human Cytomegalovirus Journal Articles	522	15.00
Immunosuppressive Therapy Journal Art.	526	20.00
Institutional Laundry Journal Articles	789	8.00
Lithium & Psychiatry Journal Articles	520	15.00
Psychosomatic Medicine Current J. Art.	788	12.00

ITEMS	Code	Unit Price
Outpatient Services Journal Articles, 2nd Ed.	797	$10.00
Outpatient Services Journal Articles, *1st Ed.*	794	8.00
Selected Papers in Inhalation Therapy	523	10.00
TYPIST HANDBOOKS		
Medical Typist's Guide for Hx & Phys.	976	4.50
Radiology Typist Handbook	981	4.50
Surgical Typist Handbook	991	4.50
Transcribers Guide to Med. Terminology	973	4.50
ESSAY Q. & A. REVIEW BOOKS		
Blood Banking Principles Rev.	339	8.00
Cardiology Review	337	10.00
Colon & Rectal Surg. Cont. Ed. Rev.	338	10.00
Neurology Review	345	10.00
Obstet. Nursing Cont. Ed. Rev.	350	5.00
Ophthalmology Review	347	10.00
Orthopedics Review	349	10.00
Psychiatry Cont. Ed. Rev.	352	10.00
Psych./Mental Hlth. Nursing Cont. Ed. Rev.	351	5.00
OTHER BOOKS		
Acid Base Homeostasis	601	4.00
Allergy Annual Review	325	12.00
Bailey & Love's Short Practice of Surgery	900	20.00
Benign & Malignant Bladder Tumors	932	15.00
Blood Groups	860	2.50
Clinical Diagnostic Pearls	730	4.50
Concentrations of Solutions	602	3.00
Critical Care Manual	983	10.00
Cryogenics in Surgery	754	24.00
Diagnosis & Treatment of Breast Lesions	748	15.00
Emergency Care Manual	984	7.50
English-Spanish Guide for Med. Personnel	721	2.50
Fundamental Orthopedics	603	4.50
Guide to Medical Reports	962	4.50
Human Anatomical Terminology	982	3.00
Illustrated Laboratory Techniques	919	10.00
Introduction to Acupuncture	753	5.00
Introduction to Blood Banking	975	8.00
Introduction to the Clinical History	729	3.00
Math for Med Techs	964	7.00
Multilingual Guide for Medical Personnel	961	2.50
Neoplasms of the Gastrointestinal Tract	736	20.00
Neurophysiology Study Guide	600	7.00
Outpatient Hemorrhoidectomy Lig. Tech.	752	12.50
Profiles in Surgery, Gynec. & Obstetrics	963	5.00
Radiological Physics Exam. Review	486	10.00
Skin, Heredity & Malignant Neoplasms	744	20.00
Testicular Tumors	743	20.00
Tissue Adhesives in Surgery	756	24.00
Understanding Hematology	977	8.00

Prices subject to change.